AIDS TO CLINICAL EXAMINATION

AIDS TO
CLINICAL EXAMINATION

Peter C Hayes
BMSc(Hons), MB, ChB(Hons), MRCP
Clinical Research Fellow,
Liver Unit,
King's College Hospital, London

Ronald S MacWalter
BMSc(Hons), MB, ChB(Hons), MRCP
Senior Registrar in Medicine (General Medicine
and Geriatrics),
John Radcliffe Hospital and
Radcliffe Infirmary, Oxford

CHURCHILL LIVINGSTONE
EDINBURGH LONDON MELBOURNE AND NEW YORK 1986

CHURCHILL LIVINGSTONE
Medical Division of Longman Group UK Limited

Distributed in the United States of America by Churchill
Livingstone Inc., 1560 Broadway, New York, N.Y.
10036, and by associated companies, branches and
representatives throughout the world.

First published 1986
  Reprinted 1987

ISBN 0-443-03323-4

British Library Cataloguing in Publication Data

Hayes, Peter C.
    Aids to clinical examination.
    (Aids)
    1. Physical diagnosis
    I. Title   II. MacWalker, Ronald S.
    616.07'54   RC76

Library of Congress Cataloging in Publication Data

Hayes, Peter C.
    Aids to clinical examination.

    Includes index.
    1. Physical diagnosis—Outlines, syllabi, etc.
    1. MacWalter, Ronald S.   II. Title. [DNLM: 1. Diagnosis
    —outlines. 2. Physical Examination—outlines.
    WB 18 H418a]
    RC76.H34   1986   616.07'5   85-29892

Produced by Longman Singapore Publishers Pte Ltd
Printed in Singapore

PREFACE

The intention of this book is to fill a gap in examination preparation. Examinations of clinical skill, like written examinations, require revision and this book is designed to help with this. It is written to replace the cards so often prepared by the student about how to examine a system or patient under examination settings. It is principally written to help students preparing for undergraduate 'final examinations' and those studying for such postgraduate diplomas as the MRCP. However, we hope it will prove useful to students studying for any form of clinical examination.

The structure of the book is such that the headings down the left hand side of the page can act as an aide memoir or checklist of things to look for, whilst the accompanying notes provide useful tips and explanations. This format also allows candidates to add notes to the text. It is realised that examinations of clinical skill are conducted under artificial circumstances and certain procedures normally part of clinical practice, such as the rectal examination, will not be required. They are however, included in the text for completeness. To keep each chapter as a relatively separate entity, a certain amount of repetition was necessary to avoid excessive cross referencing.

We are aware that this form of presentation lends itself better to certain systems than others, but have stuck to the same format throughout in the belief that it will encourage systematic examination.

London and Oxford,
1986

P.C.H
R.S.M

ACKNOWLEDGEMENT

We would like to acknowledge the editorial help of Professor I. A. D. Bouchier and secretarial skills of Ms Maureen Hughes.

CONTENTS

1. HANDS

INSPECTION	Hands frequently provide clues of underlying disease and should be closely inspected in all patients.
Size	The overall size should be noted and interpreted in the context of body size. Enlargement may be due to acromegaly (when they are described as spade-like), obesity, hypothyroidism, primary amyloidosis and manual work. Unilateral enlargement may be due to oedema such as occurs in venous or lymphatic obstruction and disuse (e.g. hemiplegia).
Involuntary Movement	Involuntary movement may be important diagnostically.
Coarse tremor	A coarse tremor at rest is seen in Parkinson's disease and is characteristically 'pill-rolling'.
Physiological tremor	The physiological tremor is fine and an exaggerated form may be seen in anxiety states, hyperthyroidism and alcoholism.
Benign essential tremor	The benign essential tremor has a slightly larger amplitude, occurs more commonly in the elderly and is exacerbated by changes in posture.
Intention tremor	An intention tremor occurs with voluntary movement and worsens as the end-point in the movement is reached: it is tested for in the 'finger-nose' test and is a feature of cerebellar disease (Ch. 18).
Asterixis	Asterixis is a flapping tremor, elicited by dorsiflexion of hands with the arms outstretched. It is seen in hepatic failure, uraemia, hypercapnia, congestive cardiac failure and Wernicke's encephalopathy.
Fasciculation	Fasciculation, the spontaneous firing of individual motor units, may be seen involving the small muscles of the hand. Although it occurs in normal subjects, motor neurone disease should be

considered, especially if there is associated muscle wasting.

Palms

Erythema

Palmar erythema is seen in chronic liver disease, rheumatoid arthritis, thyrotoxicosis and pregnancy.

Hyperkeratosis

Hyperkeratosis of the palms is seen in tylosis (a rare familial disorder associated with increased risk of oesophageal carcinoma).

Dupuytren's contracture

Dupuytren's contracture (palmar fascia fibrosis) occurs primarily in males and may have a higher incidence in patients with alcoholic liver disease, although this is disputed. It is also reputed to occur in association with manual work and epilepsy. It is common in otherwise normal subjects and may be familial. It typically affects the ring finger first and is usually bilateral, although frequently asymmetrical.

Skin creases

Skin creases are pale in anaemia, darkly pigmented in Addison's disease, and yellow in carotinaemia.

Cyanosis

Fingers, and nail beds in particular, are blue in cyanosis. If the hand is warm and cyanosed, central cyanosis exists (see Ch. 12).

Muscle wasting

Thenar eminence atrophy is seen in median nerve lesions (e.g. carpal tunnel syndrome) while hypothenar eminence wasting occurs with ulnar nerve lesions. Atrophy of the small muscles of the hand is seen in old age, cachexia, rheumatoid arthritis, T_1 root lesions, motor neurone disease, syringomyelia, cord compression, cervical rib, Klumpke's paralysis and cervical spondylosis.

Rashes

Rashes are unusual in the palms of the hands but occur in secondary syphilis, pompholyx and pustular psoriasis.

Nails

Clubbing

Finger clubbing is a hallmark of many diseases and an important physical sign. Five stages of clubbing are recognised:

1) Increased nail bed fluctuation; (examine with index fingers of each hand over the nail bed of the finger to be examined with the thumbs underneath).
2) Loss of nail bed angle (normally 140°).
3) Increased curvature of long axis of nail.
4) Soft tissue swelling at the ends of the finger

which when marked produces a drum-stick appearance.

5) Hypertrophic pulmonary osteoarthropathy may develop and is recognised by painful wrists and periosteal elevation demonstrated radiologically. Causes of clubbing can be divided into respiratory, which include bronchiectasis, bronchial carcinoma, mesothelioma, asbestosis, empyema, fibrosing alveolitis and non-respiratory, which include infective endocarditis, cyanotic congenital cardiac disease, atrial myxoma, hepatic cirrhosis, Crohn's disease, panproctocolitis, coeliac disease, brachial arteriovenous fistula (causes unilateral clubbing), thyrotoxicosis, dysproteinaemia (especially alpha-chain disease), pyelonephritis, syphilis, pregnancy and congenital.

Pseudo-clubbing
Resorption of the terminal phalanges may be seen in hyperparathyroidism, giving an appearance similar to finger clubbing, pseudo-clubbing.

Koilonychia
Koilonychia (spoon-shaped deformity) is seen in iron deficiency.

Leukonychia
Leukonychia (white discolouration) is seen in hypoalbuminaemia with or without liver disease.

Lindsay's nails
Lindsay's nails are the half white/half brown nails found in patients with chronic renal disease.

Splinter haemorrhages
Longitudinal splinter haemorrhages occur in infective endocarditis and after nail trauma. Transverse splinter haemorrhages are seen in trichinosis.

Onycholysis
Onycholysis, where the nail becomes detached distally from its plate, occurs in thyrotoxicosis, eczema, psoriasis and fungal infections.

Beau's lines
In severe illnesses, transverse indentations (Beau's lines) may occur. Longitudinal ridges are usually due to trauma.

Pitting
As well as causing onycholysis, psoriasis may produce pitting of nails which may be associated with arthropathy of affected fingers.

Nail bed infarcts
Nail bed infarcts indicate a vasculitic process and are seen particularly in systemic lupus erythematosus and rheumatoid disease.

Telangectasia of nail folds
In dermatomyositis and systemic lupus erythematosus telangectasia of nail folds may be seen.

Absent nails
Congenital absence of nails occurs and may be

associated with other congenital abnormalities such as absent or rudimentary patellae. Nails may also be absent because of previous trauma or nail bed infections.

Yellow nail syndrome   The triad of yellow nails, lymphatic oedema of lower limbs and sterile pleural effusion, is known as the yellow nail syndrome (cause unknown).

Blue lunulae   The lunulae may be coloured blue in Wilson's disease (hepatolenticular degeneration) due to increased copper deposition).

Nicotine staining   Heavily nicotine stained nails and fingers reflect more the habit of smoking a cigarette down to the butt rather than the number smoked per day.

Periungual fibroma   Hypertrophic nodules around nails, periungual fibroma, which may look like viral warts, are associated with tuberous sclerosis.

Fungal infections   Chronic fungal infections produce atrophic nails as in familial hypoparathyroidism.

Other lesions

Scabies   Red excoriated lesions, especially at the finger web area, are seen with scabies infections; the burrows are characteristic.

Joints (see Ch. 19)

Rheumatoid arthritis   Rheumatoid arthritis results in synovitis of the metacarpophalangeal joints, with filling of the hollow between metacarpal heads when the fingers are flexed and synovial swelling of extensor tendon sheaths. Tendon tears produce 'swan neck' and 'buttonairre' deformities. Swelling of the proximal interphalangeal joints produces spindle-shaped deformity (Haygarth nodes). At the wrists marked deformity may exist. Carpal tunnel syndrome may co-exist and is due to synovial hypertrophy.

Osteoarthrosis   Heberden's nodes occur at the distal interphalangeal joints in familial generalised osteoarthrosis. Bouchard's nodes occur at proximal interphalangeal joints. The 'square hand' deformity is due to involvement of thumb carpometacarpal joint. A gross but painless osteoarthrosis (Charcot's joint) may be seen in the hand in leprosy and wrist (elbow and shoulder) in syringomyelia.

Gout   Gout produces an asymmetrical pattern of arthritis with tophaceous swelling in relation to joints. The helix of the ear should also be inspected for tophi.

Pseudohypopara-thyroidism	The hand in pseudohypoparathyroidism has a characteristic appearance with shortening of the fourth metacarpal which is more readily apparent when a fist is made.

PALPATION

Osler's nodes	The finger pulps should be palpated to identify Osler's nodes which are exquisitely tender nodules and occur in infective endocarditis.
Joint tenderness	All joints should be tested for tenderness either individually or with a squeeze test examining rows of joints, being careful not to hurt the patient.
Hypertrophic pulmonary arthropathy	Tenderness around the wrist associated with finger clubbing occurs in hypertrophic pulmonary osteoarthropathy.
Passive joint movement	All joints should be put through a full range of passive movement, being careful not to cause pain. Also note whether joint crepitus occurs with movement.
Active joint movement and power	Assess grip strength and power of extension at wrist and fingers and small muscles of hand.
Median nerve	The median nerve supplies the lateral two lumbricals, opponens pollicis, abductor pollicis brevis and flexor pollicis brevis (mnemonic LOAF). The abductor pollicis brevis is tested by straight raising of the thumb vertically with the back of hand flat on a table.
Ulnar nerve	The ulnar nerve supplies all the other small muscles of the hand. An ulnar nerve lesion below the elbow produces clawing of fourth and fifth fingers. Test for joint hyper-extension at the metacarpophalangeal joints and assess abduction and adduction of the fingers. Weakness of adductor pollicis produces Froment's sign which is detected by applying traction to a sheet of paper held between the patient's thumb and clenched fist of both hands. Weakness of the adductor pollicis cause flexion of the distal phalynx of the thumb (Froment's sign).
Radial nerve	A radial nerve lesion causes wrist drop with weakness of triceps, extensor carpiradialis, extensor digitalis and extensor pollicis longus. Weakness of the extensors also produces considerable weakness of flexors as the antagonists which are necessary for stability are removed.

Sensation Abnormal sensation may be demonstrable in the hands. Two main patterns of sensory loss are recognised — those involving segmental and those involving peripheral nerves (see Fig. 1.1).

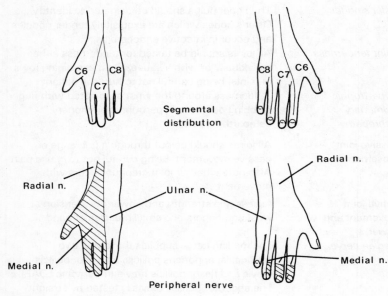

Fig. 1.1 Innervation of the hand.

2. FACE

INSPECTION

Shape — The shape of the face is important.

Cheeks — Drawn-in cheeks are seen in cancer cachexia and partial lipodystrophy. Fullness of the face may be due to obesity, Cushing's syndrome, acute glomerulonephritis, parotid swelling (as in mumps, parotitis, parotid tumours), and superior vena caval obstruction.

Bossing — Frontal bossing may be seen in rickets, congenital syphilis and sickle cell anaemia.

Swelling — Swelling of part of the face, with erythema and a sharp margin of demarcation, is seen in erysipelas while angioneurotic oedema and contact dermatitis (e.g. to drugs or eye make-up) may cause marked localised facial swelling.

Colour — The colour of the complexion is worth noting.

Pallor — Pallor is seen in anaemia, vasoconstriction, malnutrition and panhypopituitarism.

Vitiligo — Localised depigmentation as vitiligo may suggest an underlying autoimmune disorder or be idiopathic.

Albinism
Pigmentation — Total failure of pigment production is seen in albinism. Melanin pigmentation may indicate racial origin. Increased pigmentation is seen in Addison's disease, haemachromatosis, primary biliary cirrhosis and renal failute.

Chloasma — Chloasma—patchy pigmentation over forehead and around eyes—may occur in pregnancy or be due to the oral contraceptive pill.

Pigmented lesions — Pigmented lesions may be benign, such as freckles, simple naevi and seborrhoeic keratoses (greasy, warty lesions associated with increased age), or malignant, such as malignant melanoma, which may bleed or ulcerate.

Jaundice	Jaundice (see Ch. 13).
Plethora	Plethora may reflect outdoor occupation, polycythaemia or carcinoid syndrome. A malar flush may be seen in mitral stenosis and Cushing's syndrome, whilst a 'peaches and cream' appearance is seen in hypothyroidism (excess carotene gives yellowish tinge). The butterfly rash of discoid and systemic lupus erythematosus must be distinguished from facial plethora. Easy flushing is seen in acne rosacea and the carcinoid syndrome, while erythema may affect the face in l'homme rouge which may be associated with an underlying lymphoproliferative disease.

Emotional State
Agitation
Apathy

The emotional state should be noted. Agitation is seen in anxiety, mania and hyperthyroidism, while apathy is typical of depression and hypothyroidism.

Lack of expression
Lack of facial expression due to poverty of movement is seen in Parkinsonism.

Emotional lability
Emotional lability may complicate cerebrovascular accidents, especially when pseudobulbar palsy is also present.

Euphoria
Cheerfulness
Frank euphoria is sometimes seen in multiple sclerosis, while cheerfulness in the face of apparent adversity may be a sign of hysteria.

Hair
Frontal balding
Frontal balding is common in males but is a characteristic feature of dystrophia myotonica.

Alopecia
Patchy hair loss (alopecia) is seen in alopecia areata (characteristic 'exclamation-mark' hairs—normal width at the tip and narrow at the base—are found at the margins during the active phase), excessive hair-pulling (trichotillomania), secondary to cytotoxic drugs and scarring alopecia secondary to systemic lupus erythematosus, scleroderma, lichen planus, and severe fungal and bacterial infections.

Thinning
Generalised thinning of the hair may be seen in Cushing's syndrome and hypothyroidism.

Coarsening
Coarsening of the hair is also a feature of hypothyroidism.

Hirsutism
Hirsutism may be seen with adrenal lesions— adrenal tumours, Cushing's syndrome and congenital adrenal hyperplasia, be drug induced (e.g. minoxidil) or associated with ovarian lesions—

	arrhenoblastoma and polycystic ovaries. More commonly, however, it is familial, racial or idiopathic.
Lack of facial hair	Lack of facial hair is seen in hypogonadism, whilst regression of facial hair may occur in hypopituitarism.
Skin	Examination of the facial skin may show lesions associated with underlying disease or it may be involved with primary skin disease.
Facial rashes	Facial rashes are common and must be identified.
SLE	In systemic lupus erythematosus a scaly erythematous rash with typical batswing distribution over cheeks and bridge of nose occurs with scarring and atrophy.
Dermatomyositis	A heliotrope rash, especially over the eyelids, temples and cheeks (but also on the knuckles) may occur in dermatomyositis.
Acne rosacea	Acne rosacea occurs typically over the cheeks and nose and is erythematous with pustules and telangiectasia.
Carcinoid	Flushing is a feature of carcinoid syndrome; this may progress to persistent redness.
Perioral dermatitis	An erythematous papular eruption around the mouth, perioral dermatitis, may be seen in young women.
Acne vulgaris	Acne vulgaris with its characteristic folliculitis, pustule formation, comedones and excess sebum secretion, affects the face, neck, shoulders and chest in adolescence, but is also associated with the oral contraceptive pill, Cushing's syndrome and phenytoin use.
Seborrhoeic dermatitis	Seborrhoeic dermatitis is common and affects flexural areas, nasolabial fold and causes scaliness of the eyebrows.
Atopic eczema	Atopic eczema is usually intensely pruritic and scratch-marks may be seen as well as the exuding patches involving the cheeks, ears and scalp, which may progress to lichenification.
Psoriasis	Psoriatic plaques rarely occur on the face but are sometimes seen around the scalp margin, eyes, nose and ears.
Drugs	Drugs may cause any type of rash, although erythematous maculopapular types are common.
Stevens-Johnson syndrome	Stevens-Johnson syndrome, cutaneous erythema multiforme with ulceration of mucous membranes,

may be associated with drug use (e.g. penicillin and sulphonamides), but may also occur in bacterial and viral infections.

Light exposure
SLE
Polymorphic light eruption
Porphyrias

Rashes in light exposed areas are seen in systemic lupus erythematosus, polymorphic light eruption (rashes of various types), and the porphyrias. In porphyria cutanea tarda and porphyria variegata bullous eruptions may be noted; in erythropoietic protoporphyria pock-marking is seen while in erythropoietic porphyria, bullous destructive lesions are noted together with deformed and reddened teeth.

Pemphigus

Pemphigoid

Pemphigus may affect the face and mouth. The bullous lesions strip on pressure (Nikolski's sign) and heal are intra-epidermal, while pemphigoid has tense, large, blisters which are sub-epidermal and may be associated with underlying malignancy.

Dermatitis herpetiformis

Dermatitis herpetiformis — clusters of small, pruritic blisters (also on shoulders, lumbosacral area, elbows and knees) may be associated with coeliac disease.

Blisters

Blisters can be due to heat induced trauma and drug overdose (e.g. phenobarbitone) where pressure areas tend to be affected.

Toxic epidermal necrolysis

Toxic epidermal necrolysis, due to staphylococcal infection, is characterised by large blisters and crusting.

Furuncles

Furuncles (boils) are due to staphylococcal infection of hair follicles. They occur more frequently in diabetics.

Impetigo

Impetigo is a spreading infection of the epidermis common in children.

Syphilis

A primary syphilitic chancre may rarely be seen on the lips or in the mouth, while snail track ulcers of the mouth and a maculopapular rash are seen in secondary syphilis.

Lupus vulgaris

Lupus vulgaris, cutaneous tuberculosis, produces erythematous, hypertrophic, ulcerative lesions which may erode and scar. A glass-slide applied over the lesion produces an 'apple-jelly' appearance.

Lupus pernio

Lupus pernio are raised bluish-red plaques found particularly over the nose in sarcoidosis.

Leprosy

In lepromatous leprosy, nodular granulomatous lesions on the face are seen (leonine facies) while in tuberculoid leprosy, lesions may be hypopigmented and anaesthetic.

Ringworm	Ringworm may affect the scalp and face. On the scalp affected hairs are broken off leaving the scalp scaled and inflamed. Similar lesions may be seen on the face.
Candida	Candida albicans infection may cause angular cheilitis (associated with poorly-fitting dentures and vitamin deficiency), and white adherent plaques in the mouth (thrush).
Pityriasis versicolor	Pityriasis versicolor, due to the microorganism *Malasezzia furfur*, produces a scaly rash with areas of depigmentation.
Molluscum contagiosum Warts	Molluscum contagiosum, cream coloured umbilicated globular nodules and warts are caused by viral infections.
Herpes simplex	Herpes simplex, the familiar vesicular crusting cold sores, reflects secondary recrudescence of dominant infection often associated with debility or pneumonia and may be extensive in immunosuppressed patients. The primary infection itself may be severe with stomatitis and pharyngitis.
Herpes zoster	The maculovesicular rash of herpes zoster (shingles) may affect part of the distribution of the trigeminal nerve with pain and parasthesiae and, rarely, motor disturbance. The Ramsay-Hunt syndrome consists of facial palsy due to herpes zoster infection of geniculate ganglion associated with skin lesions in the external auditory meatus.
Spider naevi	Spider naevi may be seen in liver disease, pregnancy and rheumatoid arthritis (see Ch. 8).
Telangiectases	Telangiectases are seen in systemic sclerosis and hereditary haemorrhagic telangiectasia.
Cavernous haemangiomas Capillary haemangioma	Cavernous haemangiomas (strawberry naevi) are nodular and resolve spontaneously while capillary haemangioma (port-wine stain) remains and may be associated with a meningeal haemangioma (Sturge-Weber syndrome).
Adenoma sebaceum	Adenoma sebaceum are hamartomas of connective tissue and should suggest tuberous sclerosis.
Lentigines	Pigmented lentigines are seen in Peutz-Jegher's syndrome.
Melanotic freckle	The melanotic freckle, a solitary flat dark lesion which spreads slowly, is seen in the elderly and may progress to malignant melanoma.
Malignant melanoma	Malignant melanomas may be pigmented, nodular,

ulcerating lesions which may bleed or crust. They may however, be entirely amelanotic.

Solar keratoses
Solar keratoses, small irregular scaly warty plaques, are seen in fair-skinned people exposed to excessive sunlight.

Basal cell carcinoma
Basal cell carcinomas (rodent ulcers) usually have a rolled-edge and destructive centre and are associated with excess sunlight exposure. They may be seen as part of Gorlin's syndrome (with palmar pits, mandibular cysts and central nervous system tumours).

Kerato-acanthomas
Kerato-acanthomas are rapidly growing warty lesions with a central horny plug seen on light exposed areas and which are sometimes difficult to distinguish from squamous cell carcinomas.

Squamous cell carcinoma

Metastases
Deposits of metastatic carcinoma are sometimes found on the face or scalp.

Xanthalasma
See Chapter 3.

Nose

Rhinophyma
Inspection of the nose may reveal rhinophyma, where the nose is enlarged, red and bulbous in the late stages of acne rosacea.

Destruction of nasal cartilage
Destruction of nasal cartilage is seen in tertiary syphilis, Wegner's granulomatosis, lupus vulgaris, leprosy and chronic relapsing polychondritis.

Deformation
Deformation is often due to old trauma.

Discharge
A purulent discharge is seen in chronic sinusitis (consider Kartagener's syndrome) whilst a serous discharge occurs in hay fever and coryzal illnesses.

Ears

Gouty tophi
White nodules on the helix of the ear, gouty tophi, are due to deposition of sodium biurate crystals (do not confuse with Darwin's tubercle, a normal variant). Dusky pigmentation of the cartilage of the ear is seen in alkaptonuria.

Darwin's tubercle

Alkaptonuria

PALPATION

Temporal arteries
The temporal arteries are frequently tender in temporal arteritis.

Swellings
Any swelling should be palpated and its nature, size and associated lymphadenopathy (if any) identified (see Ch. 5).

Eyes
See Chapter 3.

PERCUSSION

Percussion of the face and head has limited application.

Chvostek's sign

Tapping over the facial nerve anterior to the ear in hypocalcaemia may produce twitching of facial muscles, especially the upper lip (Chvostek's sign).

Percussive auscultation

Percussive auscultation of the skull, where the forehead is percussed whilst different areas of the skull are listened to, has been proposed as a useful method of detecting extradural haematomas. In children with raised intracranial pressure, a 'cracked pot' note occurs on percussion.

AUSCULTATION

Auscultation over the eyeball and head may disclose bruits due to arteriovenous malformations.

Table 2.1   Typical facial appearances in some conditions with certain associated signs.

Condition	Facial Appearance	Other Signs
Down's syndrome	Round face Prominent epicanthic folds Low nasal bridge Large fissured tongue	Simian crease Incurved little finger Mental retardation
Hypothyroidism	Puffy face Coarsened features Coarse dry hair	Hoarse voice Bradycardia Delayed tendon jerk relaxation
Hyperthyroidism	Anxious, staring (eye signs) Sweating	Tachycardia Tremor (clubbing, pretibial myxoedema)

Cushing's syndrome	Round moon face
	Plethora
		'Lemon on sticks'
		  apearance
		Buffalo hump, Striae
		  (Hirsutism)

Addison's disease	Hyperpigmented	Pigmented palmar crease and buccal mucosa

Acromegaly	Coarse features
	Prominent jaw, nose,
	  lower lip
		Large hands and feet
		  (Bitemporal hemianopia)

Paget's disease	Increased skull size Platybasia (cranial nerve palsies)	
Parkinson's disease	Expressionless face Excess sebum secretion Drooling of saliva	Tremor Rigidity Akinesia
Dystrophia myotonica	Frontal baldness Wasted facial muscles Transverse smile	Sternomastoid wasting Cataract

Facial Palsy (LMN)
  (Bell's Palsy)
	Facial weakness on
	  affected side
	Affects forehead muscles
		Cannot close eye

Scleroderma
  (Systemic Sclerosis)
	Tightening of skin over
	  nose and around mouth
	Telangiectases
		Sclerodactyly, Raynaud's
		  (calcinosis—CRST)

3. EYES

INSPECTION

General

Proptosis

The eyes should be inspected from the front, sides and from above to avoid missing mild proptosis. From the front particular attention should be paid to apparent size and symmetry. Slight differences in the palpebral fissure should be looked for and an assessment made as to whether lid retraction in one eye or ptosis of the other is responsible for the asymmetry.

Lid retraction

Lid retraction is usually bilateral and is recognised when a rim of sclera is present above the iris. Causes of lid retraction include thyrotoxicosis and situations associated with sympathetic overactivity, e.g. left ventricular failure.

Ptosis

Causes of ptosis can be divided into muscular, such as myasthenia gravis and dystrophia myotonica or neurological, such as Horner's syndrome. A complete ptosis accompanies third cranial nerve palsy.

Lid lag

Lid lag is frequently associated with lid retraction and should be looked for by asking the patient to stare at the examiner's finger as it is moved slowly up and down. The upper eyelid is delayed in following the downward movement of the eye. This is a useful confirmatory sign in thyrotoxicosis.

Exophthalmos

Exophthalmos is recognised when a rim of sclera is seen both above and below the iris. An exophthalmometer should be used to measure the degree of exophthalmos. It may be unilateral as with periorbital neoplasms or infections and carotico-cavernous sinus fistulae. Although cavernous sinus thrombosis may cause bilateral exophthalmos, the commonest cause by far is thyrotoxicosis. It should be remembered that there may be marked asymmetry in the severity of exophthalmos in each eye and that there may be no other signs of thyroid overactivity present.

Eyelids

Blinking

The frequency of blinking should be noted. In Parkinsonism and in blind patients it may be infrequent.

Ectropion

Ectropion, or eversion of the lower lid, is common in the elderly, but is also associated with chronic facial palsy.

Entropion

Entropion or inversion of the lower lid complicates severe blepharitis and trachoma.

Hordeolum

Infection around an eyelash, a hordeolum or sty, is common; the other swelling of the lid which

Chalazion

involves the meibomian glands is the chalazion.

Dacryoadenitis

Inflammation of the lacrimal glands, dacryoadenitis, produces swelling in the upper outer aspect of the eyelid. Bilateral dacryoadenitis occurs with sarcoidosis, syphilis, tuberculosis and leukaemia.

Periorbital and lid oedema

Periorbital and lid oedema may occur in association with local infection and be a feature of hypothyroidism, cardiac failure and nephrotic syndrome.

Xanthelasma

Xanthelasma, cholesterol deposits in the eyelids, occur with chronic obstructive jaundice, diabetes mellitus, myxoedema, nephrotic syndrome and familial hypercholesterolaemia.

Conjunctiva

Conjunctivitis

Injection of the conjunctival blood vessels reflects conjunctival inflammation. It is usually bilateral and causes include bacterial and viral infection, foreign body (unilateral), allergies, sarcoidosis, tuberculosis and Stevens-Johnson syndrome.

Chemosis

Chemosis, oedema of the conjunctiva, occurs in severe infections, cavernous sinus thrombosis, retro-orbital tumours and with severe exophthalmos.

Sclera

Jaundice

The sclera should be examined for jaundice.

Blue discolouration

Blue discolouration of the sclera in adults occurs in osteogenesis imperfecta. In the elderly, choroidal pigment may be visible through the sclera.

Episcleritis	Occasionally systemic disorders such as rheumatoid disease and sarcoidosis may cause episcleritis. In rheumatoid disease this may proceed to ulceration and perforation of the sclera.
Iris	The iris should be inspected with a bright light at the same time as testing the pupillary reflexes.
Brushfield spots	Brushfield spots, small white areas are seen in Down's syndrome.
Iritis	Iritis is characterised by injection of the circumcorneal blood vessels. This may occur acutely due to bacterial infection or Reiter's syndrome or be chronic as in syphilis, tuberculosis, sarcoidosis, sympathetic ophthalmitis, and ankylosing spondylitis.
Uveitis	With uveitis that affects primarily the choroid, the eye is painless and the patient complains only of deteriorating vision. Uveitis occurs in sarcoidosis, ankylosing spondylitis, ulcerative colitis, Reiter's syndrome, rheumatoid arthritis, tuberculosis and syphilis.

Cornea

Keratitis	Keratitis is painful and associated with a circumcorneal injection, which may be slight.
Corneal ulceration	It may progress to corneal ulceration which may be marginal, such as in staphylococcal infection, or central, related to a foreign body, abrasion or dendritic ulcer. Congenital syphilis is associated with bilateral keratitis.
Kerato-conjunctivitis sicca	Abnormal dryness of the eyes, seen in Sjögren's syndrome, may also cause keratitis (kerato-conjunctivitis sicca).
Arcus cornealis	A white ring at the outer margin of the cornea, the so-called arcus cornealis or senilis, is commoner with increasing age: its presence in younger patients should raise the possibility of hypercholesterol-aemia.
Kayser-Fleischer rings	Kayser-Fleischer rings are seen in Wilson's disease (see Ch. 13).
Calcification	Bands or flecks of calcification may be found in association with chronic hypercalcaemia.

Pupils

Size/shape/symmetry/ reactivity	The pupils should be inspected with a bright light and their size, shape, symmetry and reactivity to

light noted. The light reflex is tested by shining a bright light from the side, avoiding the front which may provoke a convergence reaction. Both direct and consensual reactions should be tested in both eyes.

Argyll Robertson   The Argyll Robertson pupil is small and irregular and reacts to accommodation but not to light.

Holmes-Adie   The Holmes-Adie pupil, on the other hand, is large and reacts sluggishly to light and accommodation. It may be associated with absent tendon reflexes, and is said to occur more commonly in women.

Horner's syndrome   In Horner's syndrome, the pupil is constricted and associated with partial ptosis, enophthalmos and ipsilateral anhydrosis. It is due to a lesion in the cervical sympathetic chain.

Constriction   Miosis (constricted pupils) is seen in iritis, opiate use, pontine lesions and with corneal or conjunctival irritation.

Dilatation   Bilateral dilatation of the pupils is frequently due to anxiety. Unilateral pupillary dilatation may be due to an amblyopic eye, third cranial nerve lesion, acute glaucoma, Holmes-Adie pupil, mydriatic drops and multiple sclerosis.

Cataracts   Cataracts, although best seen with the ophthalmoscope, are frequently visible using the torch, shining the beam of light tangentially.

Ophthalmoscopy   Although ophthalmoscopy is a technique of inspection, it is usually left to the end of the examination (see p. 20).

Eye Movements   Eye movements should be checked with the patient's head held steady with one hand, using the other as a moving target on which the patient fixes attention. Movement should be checked in vertical and horizontal planes. The corneal light reflections should be watched as their relative positions alter if one eye moves abnormally.

Diplopia   Ask specifically about diplopia and in what direction it is maximal. The eye responsible for the more peripheral image is the affected eye.

Pain   Pain, associated with eye movement may suggest optic neuritis.

Nystagmus   Nystagmus should be looked for also during this procedure. For this reason, the target finger must be held at least 50 cm from the patient's eyes and the extremes of lateral gaze avoided. Nystagmus that is not maintained for 5 seconds is probably not significant (commenting on 'a few nystagmoid jerks' should be avoided in examinations). If nystagmus is identified, it should be described as pendular, rotary or jerking. If jerking, the direction of the rapid phase is used to describe the direction of nystagmus, and the direction of gaze at which it is maximal noted.

Vertigo   Associated symptoms such as vertigo should be recorded.

Ataxic nystagmus   Ataxic nystagmus (internuclear ophthalmoplegia) is characterised by nystagmus of the abducted eye and restricted adduction of the medial looking eye. It is relatively common in examinations and is nearly always due to multiple sclerosis.

Conjugate deviation   Failure of upward conjugate deviation can occur in disorders of the extra-pyramidal system (e.g. progressive supranuclear palsy and Parkinson's disease), but also can occur in Alzheimer's disease and in old age.

Visual Fields

Confrontation   The visual fields should be assessed by confrontation. The examiner should sit opposite the patient, approximately 1 metre away, and cover one of their eyes. The patient should fix on the examiner's opposite eye. The peripheral visual fields are then assessed by moving a target into the field of vision from upper and lower, medial and lateral quadrants. The patient's visual field is checked against the examiners. The moving target used is usually the examiner's index finger although use of a red and white hat pin is more accurate.

Menace reflex   In subjects who cannot cooperate with this test (e.g. drowsy or unconscious subjects), the menace reflex can be useful and is elicited by the examiner bringing his hand rapidly towards the patient's eye from their lateral field of vision and reflex blinking identified. Common visual field abnormalities are described in Table 3.1.

Visual Acuity

Print   The visual acuity can be assessed simply at the bedside by asking the patient to read newsprint of various sizes with each eye separately. The patient should wear their glasses if these are usually worn

Table 3.1   Visual field abnormalities.

Field Loss	Site of Lesion
Total field loss from one eye	Retina or optic nerve
Bitemporal hemianopia	Optic chiasma
Non-congruous hemianopia	Optic tract
Upper homonymous quadrantanopia	Optic radiation (temporal)
Lower homonymous quadrantanopia	Optic radiation (parietal)
Homonymous hemianopia with macular sparing	Occipital cortex
Inattention hemianopia	Parietal lobe
Enlarged blind spot	Early papilloedema
Concentric constriction of field	Late papilloedema
Central scotoma (+ poor acuity)	Papillitis

Finger and light recognition	for reading. If the acuity is very poor, the ability to count fingers or perceive light should be checked.
AUSCULTATION	Auscultation over the closed eye may reveal a bruit and should always be performed in patients with proptosis. In carotico-cavernous fistulae, pulsating exophthalmos is associated with a systolic bruit.
PALPATION	The intraocular pressure can be assessed approximately (with practice) by eliciting fluctuation over the downward looking eye.
OPHTHALMOSCOPY	Ophthalmoscopy is usually carried out last. This examination is important and proficiency comes with practice. For a complete examination of the fundus, mydriatic drops must be used.
Cornea	Initially the cornea must be inspected with the ophthalmoscope held a few centimetres from the eye.
Opacities	Opacities in the cornea and anterior chamber, lens and vitreous will appear as black spots. Thereafter the instrument is brought close to the patient's eye and a suitable lens selected to bring the retina into focus. The following should be specifically inspected.
Optic disc	a) the optic disc, checking its size, shape, colour, margins and physiological cup

Table 3.2 Fundal changes in common conditions.

Condition	Features	Causes

Papilloedema	Hyperaemia of disc
	Obliteration of cup
	Congestion of veins and
	  loss of pulsation
	Haemorrhages radiating
	  from disc
		Malignant hypertension
		Raised IC pressure
		Central retinal vein
		  obstruction
		CO_2 retention

Papillitis	Similar to papilloedema	Retrobulbar neuritis
Optic atrophy	Pale disc, blurred edge Pale disc, sharp edge	Secondary to papilloedema Retrobulbar neuritis Optic nerve pressure Diabetes mellitus Retinal vein occlusion

Myelinated nerve fibres	Streaky irregular white
	  patches adjacent to disc
	  margin
		Normal variant

Angioid streaks	Streaks across retina resembling blood vessels	Paget's disease Pseudoxanthoma elasticum Hyperphosphataemia Acromegaly

Diabetes mellitus
  (Background)
 	
  (Proliferative)
	Venous dilatation and
	  tortuosity
	Microaneurysms
	Blot haemorrhages
	Soft exudates (cotton-wool
	  spots)
	New vessel formation
	Vitreous haemorrhage
	Retinal detachment
	Retinitis proliferans
		Both insulin dependent and
		  non insulin dependent
		  diabetes mellitus

Hypertension	Tortuous arteries
	a-v nipping
	Varying vessel calibre
	Flame haemorrhages
	Hard exudates
	Papilloedema
		Hypertension—
		  (Grades I & II)
		
		  (Grade III)
		
		  (Grade IV)

Anaemia	Pale background, engorged
	  blood vessels, flame-
	  shaped haemorrhages;
	  wooly exudates
		Severe anaemia of any
		  cause especially
		  pernicious anaemia, and
		  leukaemia

Blood vessels	b) retinal blood vessels, looking particularly at arterio-venous crossings and vessel calibre and tortuosity
Retina	c) background retina, looking for pigmentary abnormalities, exudates, haemorrhages and new vessels

Periphery

d) periphery, looking for pigmentary changes and retinal tears

Macula

e) the macular region, which is inspected last by asking the patient to look straight at the light. It is darker in colour and free of blood vessels. The central depression, the fovea, should be identified. Abnormalities in this region are especially important and affect visual acuity. Familiarity with typical hypertensive and diabetic retinopathies is essential for examinations. Common fundal changes are shown in Table 3.2.

4. CRANIAL NERVES

I Olfactory

Anosmia

The sense of smell should be tested with various scents (e.g. coffee, peppermint, vanilla), testing each nostril separately. Anosmia may be due to a frontal lobe tumour, meningioma, skull fracture, or Kallman's syndrome.

II, III, IV & VI

The testing of these cranial nerves is covered in Chapter 3.

V Trigeminal

Masseter

Inspect the muscles of mastication and palpate the masseters when the patient's teeth are clenched.

Pterygoid

Ask the patient to open and close jaw against resistance. The jaw will move towards the side of a weakened pterygoid muscle.

Jaw jerk

The jaw jerk is brisk in upper motor neurone lesions.

Corneal reflex

The corneal reflex is a useful test as it may be impaired in trigeminal nerve damage. It must however, be tested carefully. The cornea should be lightly touched with a wisp of cotton wool, being careful to approach the eye laterally, out of the field of vision. Ask the patient if each side feels equally unpleasant (V nerve), and watch for asymmetry of eye closure in response (orbicularis oculi—VII nerve).

Sensation

Light touch and pinprick sensation should be tested comparing each side of the forehead, cheeks and jaws, thereby testing the three divisions of the trigeminal nerve.

VII Facial

Facial muscles

Voluntary contractions of the facial muscles should be examined and the two sides compared. Ask the patient to frown, raise eyebrows, wrinkle forehead, close eyes, puff out cheeks, show teeth (not 'smile' which is an emotional response) and whistle. Unilateral upper motor neurone lesions relatively spare the forehead, unlike lower motor neurone lesions.

Bell's sign   Bell's sign, an exaggerated upward movement of the eyeball on attempted eye closure, is seen in lower motor neurone lesions.

Myasthenia   Repeated testing of facial muscles may show progressive weakening in myasthenia gravis.

Sensation   Traditionally, taste sensation over the anterior two-thirds of the tongue is tested using sugar, salt, vinegar and quinine on each side of the tongue. The mouth should be rinsed between each test.
However touching the tongue with the terminals of a small transistor battery can be a good guide to loss of sensation.

Glabellar tap   The glabellar tap, repeated percussion over the root of the nose, shows attenuation of blinking in normal subjects, but not in Parkinsonism. This sign is not generally believed to be particularly accurate diagnostically.

Snout reflex   The snout reflex, puckering or protrusion of the lips, is elicited by stroking the upper lip and is positive in frontal lobe disease or bilateral facial nerve upper motor neurone lesions.

Hyperacusis   Hyperacusis occurs in geniculate ganglion lesions due to paralysis of the stapedius muscle.

VIII Auditory

Hearing   A rough assessment of hearing may be made by whispering in, or holding a ticking watch near to each ear. The opposite external meatus should be occluded by a finger during testing.

Rinne's test   Rinne's test is performed using a high-pitched (256 Hz) tuning fork initially placed near the ear and then applied to the mastoid. Air conduction is louder than bone conduction in normal subjects and in nerve deafness, bone conduction is louder in conductive deafness.

Weber's test   Weber's test is performed by applying a tuning fork to the middle of the forehead. Normally the sound is heard in the midline. It is heard on the affected side in conduction or middle ear deafness and on the unaffected side in nerve or inner ear deafness.

Auroscopy

Auroscopy of external auditory meatus looking for wax, signs of infection or a foreign body should be carried out and then the tympanic membrane inspected for perforation, redness or deformity.

VIII Vestibular

The vestibular part of the VIII nerve is usually tested only when indicated.

Nystagmus

Nystagmus should be looked for when testing eye movements. Positional nystagmus should be tested by lowering the patient's head off the bed below the horizontal and turning the head. The nystagmus produced is persistent in brain stem and cerebellar lesions but with time reduces with damage to the otolithic apparatus. (See also Ch. 18).

IX Glossopharyngeal

Gag reflex

Touching the posterior wall of the pharynx with a tongue depressor evokes the gag reflex and tests the glossopharyngeal nerve.

Palatal reflex

The palatal reflex is more pleasant for the patient and is elicited by touching each side of the palate with an orange stick in turn. Taste to posterior third of tongue is difficult to test.

X Vagus

Palatal movement

Palatal movement is assessed by asking the patient to say 'Ah'. The palate and uvula are pulled away from the weakened side.

Dysphonia

Dysphonia may be due to recurrent laryngeal nerve palsy and if present the vocal cords should be examined by indirect laryngoscopy using a laryngeal mirror.

XI Accessory

The accessory nerve is tested by assessing the power of the trapezius and sternomastoid muscles against resistance. Turning the head away from the affected side is weakened in accessory nerve palsy. Bilateral weakness of the trapezius is seen in poliomyelitis and motor neurone disease whilst weakness of the sternomastoid occurs in muscular dystrophy, dystophia myotonica and motor neurone disease.

XII Hypoglossal

The tongue resting in the mouth, should be inspected for fasciculation and wasting in lower motor neurone lesions. The tongue deviates towards the affected side on voluntary protrusion. In bilateral upper motor neurone lesions, tongue movement is sluggish. Rapid protrusion and retraction of the tongue (trombone tremor) occurs in Parkinsonism and in general paralysis of the insane. Continuous rotatory movements of the tongue are frequently drug-induced (e.g. phenothiazines).

5. NECK

INSPECTION

The general appearance of the patient should be noted, particularly for evidence of thyrotoxicosis or myxoedema. Inspection of the neck should be carried out from the front, back and both sides, in good light, with adequate exposure of the neck and shoulders.

Shape

Short neck

An abnormally short neck may indicate an underlying abnormality of the cervical spine such as the Klippel-Feil syndrome which may be associated with compression of the cervical cord.

Webbing

Webbing of the neck is a classical feature of Turner's syndrome.

Kyphosis

Kyphosis may be noted with advancing years.

Swellings

Goitre
Cysts
Salivary glands
Lymph nodes
Carotid pulse

Swellings such as goitre, branchial and thyroglossal cysts, cystic hygroma, salivary gland enlargement and lymphadenopathy should be noted. A thyroglossal cyst rises on swallowing. Expansile carotid pulsation may be seen on the right side of the neck due to a kinked carotid artery, which is related to aortic unfolding and hypertension, or an aneurysm. The abnormality on inspection may be restricted to the back of the neck, e.g. the buffalo hump of Cushing's syndrome.

Buffalo hump

Scars

Scars of thyroid and parathyroid surgery should be looked for and their age estimated; if recent, latent tetany may be demonstrated as a positive Chvostek's or Trousseau's sign. The irregular scars of scrofula may be present, particularly in the elderly and indicates past tuberculous involvement of the cervical lymph nodes.

Skin

Vitiligo

Pseudoxanthoma elasticum

The skin should be inspected for vitiligo (associated with auto-immune disease) and the 'plucked chicken' appearance of pseudoxanthoma elasticum (associated with arthropathy).

Spider naevi

Spider naevi may be prominent on the neck. A total of more than six should lead to a search for other signs of liver disease (Ch. 8).

Scleroderma

Tightening of the skin of the neck may suggest systemic sclerosis.

Jugular Venous Pulse

The jugular venous pulse (JVP) which refers to the internal jugular vein should be looked for with the patient reclining at 45° with the neck relaxed. It is seen welling up between the heads of the sternomastoid. It may or may not be pulsatile. It can be differentiated from the carotid pulse by the following characteristics: it is only rarely palpable, is biphasic, rises and falls relatively slowly and rises if pressure is applied over the vein at the base of the neck or over the abdomen (hepatojugular reflux). This latter is particularly conspicuous in tricuspid regurgitation and may be absent in hepatic vein occlusion (Budd-Chiari syndrome). The vertical height of the column of blood above the sternal angle should be measured. The JVP may not be easy to recognise when the venous pressure is grossly elevated (look for ear lobe pulsation) and may only become clearly visible when the patient is erect. A rough guide to the height of the JVP is to check the level at which the veins in the elevated arm collapse. The character of the venous pulsation should be assessed. Characteristic wave forms are shown in Figure 5.1.

Kussmaul's sign

Constrictive pericarditis

Elevation of the JVP with inspiration is known as Kussmaul's sign and occurs when there is obstruction to venous filling of the heart as occurs in constrictive pericarditis.

SVC obstruction

A non-pulsatile JVP suggests superior vena caval obstruction; associated signs include oedema of the upper body, facial plethora and distension of superficial veins over the upper chest. The direction of flow in these veins should be ascertained and is downwards (towards the umbilicus) in superior vena caval obstruction.

i) Normal

ii) Large 'v' and slow 'x' descent -
    tricuspid regurgitation

iii) Large 'a' - TS, PS, pulmonary
     hypertension. Complete heart
     block (Cannon wave)

iv) Deep 'y' descent -
    constrictive pericarditis

v) Absent 'a' — atrial fibrillation

Fig. 5.1 Characteristic jugular venous wave forms.

Muscles

Accessory muscles of respiration	Use of accessory muscles of respiration may be obvious in obstructive airways disease.
Sternomastoid wasting	Sternomastoid wasting is a hallmark of dystrophia myotonica.
Torticollis	Torticollis or wryneck may be obvious and if chronic may produce facial asymmetry. The patient should be asked to touch each shoulder in turn with both chin and ear to identify limitation of movement.
Sternomastoid tumour	In infancy a hard nodule within the sternomastoid muscle is referred to as a sternomastoid tumour.

PALPATION

Palpation of the back and sides of the neck should be performed from in front of the patient.

Thyroid Swellings

Goitre Palpation of a goitre should be bimanual and is customarily done from behind the patient, with the patient's head in a neutral or even slightly flexed position. The texture of the gland should be noted as well as its size. Confirmation of a swelling in the neck being thyroid or related to it, is done by asking the patient to swallow. (A glass of water should be provided if you ask the patient to swallow more than once.)

Grave's disease Enlargement of the gland may be diffuse (Grave's disease, auto-immune thyroiditis and simple goitre),

Carcinoma
Viral thyroiditis

or nodular (toxic nodular, late simple goitre and carcinoma).
Tenderness is characteristic of viral thyroiditis, but can be seen in auto-immune thyroiditis and carcinoma. Attachment of the gland to surrounding tissue suggests malignancy. Retrosternal extension of a goitre should be checked for by palpation in the suprasternal notch and by sternal percussion.

Subcutaneous Emphysema

The characteristic crackling sensation of subcutaneous emphysema (gas within the tissues) may be felt on palpation and is associated with trauma, most frequently a fractured rib puncturing the lung, rupture of the oesophagus, or rarely, gas gangrene.

Salivary Glands

Parotid

Parotid gland enlargement is usually bilateral in acute inflammatory conditions, most commonly mumps. They may be enlarged in diabetes mellitus and debilitated alcoholic patients. Tuberculosis, sarcoidosis, Sjögren's syndrome, syphilis and lymphoma can cause unilateral or bilateral enlargement. Unilateral parotid swelling may be due to a 'mixed' parotid tumour which can grow to considerable size. Intermittent swelling may be caused by duct calculi. The parotid duct opening, opposite the second upper molars must be examined. Reddening around the opening is seen in mumps and pus may be expressed in suppurative parotitis. Mikulicz's syndrome is characterised by enlargement of salivary and lacrimal glands and xerostomia. Parotid enlargement may be associated with a LMN VII nerve palsy, e.g. in 'mixed' parotid tumour, tuberculosis, syphilis, lymphoma, and leukaemia. Uveo-parotid syndrome is parotid enlargement, iridocyclitis with or without choroiditis.

Submandibular

Enlargement of the submandibular glands is rare, but should be checked for as swelling beneath and anterior to the angle of the jaw. Swelling that is intermittent and related to meals is due to Wharton's submandibular duct obstruction.

Lymphadenopathy

The neck should be palpated systematically. From the front palpate the back and sides of the neck.

Thereafter, sit the patient forward and continue palpation from behind: begin superiorly and examine the submandibular and tonsilar lymph nodes, continue over the anterior and posterior triangles of the neck, and conclude by palpating above the clavicles and deep to the sternoclavicular insertions of the sternomastoids. It is important to include all salivary glands and lymph nodes (see Fig. 5.2). Cervical nodes are sometimes more easily palpable when the patient performs a Valsalva manoeuvre.

Localised
Generalised
Primary
Secondary

Lymphadenopathy may be localised or generalised and generally reflects either infection or malignancy. The latter may be primary (lymphoma or leukaemia) or secondary and attention should be paid to the tongue, throat, nose and paranasal sinuses as well as more readily apparent areas when deciding the origin of the lymphadenopathy.

Troisier's sign

Enlargement of the left supraclavicular lymph nodes (Virchow's node) may indicate a carcinoma of the stomach is present (Troisier's sign).

A 10-point checklist of any swelling should be made (see below) and will assist in the interpretation of the problem. Swellings in neighbouring tissues and regional lymph nodes should be sought and usually indicates spread of infection or tumour.

10-point checklist for swellings

---

1. Size
2. Shape
3. Surface texture
4. Colour
5. Consistency
6. Margins
7. Mobility
8. Position
9. Tenderness
10. Temperature

Trachea

Deviation
Length
Tug

} See Chapter 7.

Tracheal 'tug' may be felt in airways obstruction or with a syphilitic aortic aneurysm.

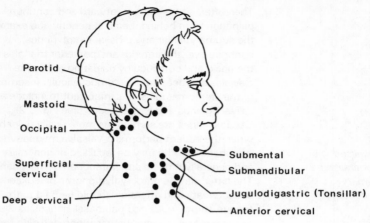

Parotid

Mastoid

Occipital

Superficial
cervical

Deep cervical

Submental

Submandibular

Jugulodigastric (Tonsillar)

Anterior cervical

Fig. 5.2   Lymph nodes of the neck.

Carotid Pulse

The carotid pulses should be palpated with the thumb (one side at a time only) and the rate, rhythm, volume and character noted (Ch. 6).

Corrigan's sign

An easily visible carotid pulsation in aortic regurgitation is known as Corrigan's sign. A visible carotid pulse may also be seen in older patients and may be due to arteriosclerosis or aneurysmal dilation. In the young, an obvious arterial pulse in the suprasternal notch should suggest coarctation of the aorta.

PERCUSSION

Retrosternal goitre

A retrosternal goitre may be identified by percussion, though percussion of the neck is not routinely carried out.

AUSCULTATION

Bruit

Goitre

A bruit may be heard over a goitre and usually indicates thyrotoxicosis as opposed to a non-toxic goitre.

Carotid
Radiated cardiac
murmurs

Vascular bruits from carotid or subclavian stenosis may be heard in the neck as may radiated cardiac murmurs, particularly aortic stenosis.

Venous hum

A venous hum may be heard above either clavicle in a sitting or reclining patient but is not heard in supine subjects. It is commoner in children. Its intensity varies with head movement and can be abolished by pressure on the neck above the stethoscope.

Subcutaneous emphysema

When subcutaneous emphysema is suspected, ausculation over the suspected area may enable crackling to be heard when crepitus is difficult to feel.

6. CARDIOVASCULAR SYSTEM

GENERAL INSPECTION	It is helpful to note general changes first.
Pallor	Pallor may suggest shock due to myocardial infarction or pulmonary embolus, or anaemia which can itself cause a tachycardia and worsening of cardiac failure, or can be due to infective endocarditis.
Dresden doll face	A pale appearance likened to a Dresden china doll's is sometimes seen with aortic stenosis.
Anxiety	An anxious appearance may suggest underlying thyrotoxicosis or phaeochromocytoma, but anxiety itself may cause a tachycardia and a raised jugular venous pressure.
Sweating	A 'cold' sweat is a common accompaniment of myocardial infarction.
Peripheral cyanosis	Cyanosis, which may be peripheral or central, (see Ch. 12) should be noted; peripheral cyanosis with cold extremities suggests a low output state while central cyanosis may be due to right-to-left cardiac shunts or cor pulmonale.
Breathlessness	Acute breathlessness may accompany a myocardial infarction, left ventricular failure or pulmonary embolus, while chronic breathlessness may suggest cor pulmonale, which is commonly secondary to chronic obstructive airways disease.
Orthopnoea	Orthopnoea, breathlessness induced by lying flat, is a sign of incipient left ventricular failure.
Face	
Mitral facies	Mitral facies, a bluish discolouration of the cheeks is seen in mitral stenosis, but is not specific to the disease. A 'peaches and cream' complexion with fullness of the face should alert one to myxoedema.
Myxoedema *Polycythaemia*	High colour of the face, sometimes with suffusion

of the conjunctivae, is seen in polycythaemia but is more often related to outdoor exposure.

Down's syndrome
The typical facial appearance of Down's syndrome should alert the examiner to the possibility of an atrial septal defect.

Head nodding
Nodding of the head in time with the arterial pulse is sometimes seen in aortic regurgitation (De Mussett's sign) and should be differentiated from titubation or Parkinsonism.

Argyll Robertson pupils
Argyll Robertson pupils are seen in tertiary syphilis and may be associated with aortic regurgitation.

Lens dislocation
High arched palate
Lens dislocation may be seen in Marfan's syndrome as may a high arched palate (also seen in supravalvular aortic stenosis).

Hands and Legs
Careful examination of the hands may also provide helpful clues.

Finger clubbing
Finger clubbing is seen in cyanotic congenital heart disease and infective endocarditis or may suggest underlying chest disease (see Ch. 7).

Splinters
Osler's nodes
Janeway lesions
Splinter haemorrhages are seen in infective endocarditis as are Osler's nodes (tender palpalable nodules in the pulps of the fingertips), Janeway lesions (palpable purpuric spots on the palm) and necrotic lesions due to emboli.

Rheumatoid deformity
Rheumatoid deformity of the hands and rheumatoid nodules around the elbows should alert the examiner to cardiac involvement such as pericarditis and cardiomyopathy.

Scleroderma
Atrophy of the fingertips with or without infarction should suggest systemic sclerosis which may also affect the heart.

Capillary pulsations
Exaggerated nail bed capillary pulsations elucidated by slight pressure distally over the nails is seen in aortic regurgitation.

Arachnodactyly
Arachnodactyly is seen in Marfan's syndrome which is associated with aortic regurgitation, mitral regurgitation, aortic dissection and conduction abnormalities.

Xanthomas
Tendon xanthomas, as well as xanthelasma and arcus cornealis should be noted as they occur in hypercholesterolaemia.

Oedema
Peripheral oedema over both feet and ankles is typical of congestive cardiac failure, but also occurs in association with hypoalbuminaemia and inferior

vena caval obstruction. In congestive cardiac failure and hypoproteinaemia, fluid tends to collect in the most dependent part of the body. Sacral oedema therefore must be looked for in bed-bound patients.

Deep venous thrombosis
Swelling also occurs with a deep venous thrombosis with associated signs of erythema, tenderness, dilated superficial veins and increased skin temperature.

Neck
Inspection of the neck, and the jugular venous pressure in particular, is conventionally performed after palpating the peripheral pulse (see Ch. 5).

Chest

Café au lait
Café au lait patches can occur in infective endocarditis and neurofibromatosis.

Pectus excavatum
Pectus excavatum or funnel chest deformity is relatively common and can cause displacement of the heart.

Pectus carinatum
Pectus carinatum or pigeon chest and prominent Harrison's sulci are seen in rickets.

Left parasternal impulse
A left parasternal impulse is sometimes visible in right ventircular hypertrophy.

Apex beat
The apex beat can be seen sometimes in thin individuals and is more prominent with hyperdynamic states.

Kyphoscoliosis
Kyphoscoliotic deformities of the spine can cause displacement of the heart and cardiac failure, while the rigid kyphotic back of ankylosing spondylitis should alert to the possibility of aortic regurgitation.

Straight back
The rigid straight spine of the straight back syndrome is associated with a parasternal systolic murmur.

Abdomen

Ascites
Abdominal distention due to ascites may occur in severe congestive cardiac failure and constrictive pericarditis.

Aortic pulsation
Although pulsation in the upper abdomen is common in healthy, thin subjects, it may be obvious in patients with an aortic aneurysm.

PALPATION

Skin temperature
The skin temperature, especially of the hands and feet, should be noted and an assessment made of the peripheral circulation.

Capillary filling	The speed of return of capillary filling following blanching produced by applying pressure over the skin of the fingers, toes and earlobes is frequently used to assess the adequacy of the peripheral
Peripheral pulses	circulation, as well as checking the presence of peripheral pulses.

Rate

Normally the radial pulse is checked first and the rate determined.

Sinus bradycardia

Physiological variation in the heart rate is 60–100 beats per minute. A slower heart rate may be due to a sinus bradycardia (40–60) which occurs in athletes, post-myocardial infarction, hypothyroidism, hypothermia and raised intra-cranial pressure.

Complete heart block

In complete heart block the rate is usually slower (30–45) and associated with Cannon waves seen in the jugular venous pulse. It may complicate myocardial infarction and cardiomyopathy or be drug-induced or idiopathic.

Sinus tachycardia

A rapid heart rate may be due to a sinus tachycardia (>100) which may be seen in anxiety, cardiac failure, fever, anaemia, thyrotoxicosis, and children, or to a

Supraventricular tachycardia

supraventricular tachycardia (120–200) which is frequently paroxysmal and idiopathic but may be due to thyrotoxicosis, ischaemic heart disease, excess tobacco and caffeine, or pre-excitation syndromes (Wolff-Parkinson-White and Lown-Ganong-Levine). Carotid sinus massage may restore

Atrial flutter

sinus rhythm in supraventricular tachycardia. Atrial flutter with 2:1 block (150) may slow in a stepwise fashion during carotid pressure (150→100→75) and is associated with ischaemic heart disease, thyrotoxicosis and digoxin toxicity.

Rhythm

The rhythm should also be determined from the radial pulse—the rhythms described above are all regular.

Irregular
Sinus arrhythmia
Ventricular ectopics

Irregularities may be due to sinus arrhythmia (variation with respiration—common in young adults) or multiple ventricular ectopic beats (seen in ischaemia, thyrotoxicosis and cardiomyopathy), in which case, the rhythm may become regular after exercise.

Coupled beats
Dropped beats

Coupled beats (bigemini) are characteristic of digoxin toxicity whilst true 'dropped beats' occur in second degree heart block.

Atrial flutter	Atrial flutter with variable block may be
Atrial fibrillation	intermittently irregular while atrial fibrillation, which complicates hypertension, ischaemia, rheumatic heart disease and thyrotoxicosis, or more rarely, pulmonary embolus, alcoholic cardiomyopathy and pericarditis, is 'irregularly irregular'. Atrial fibrillation does not become regular with exercise. A pulse deficit between radial and apical rates may be noted.
Ventricular tachycardia	The pulse in ventricular tachycardia (120 – 200) is irregular and frequently feeble. No pulse is felt in
Ventricular fibrillation	either ventricular fibrillation or asystole.
Radial pulse	An absent radial pulse may be a congenital abnormality or due to arterial embolism or a Blalock shunt.
Character and Volume	The character and volume of the pulse is best assessed at the carotid artery, using the thumb.
Plateau pulse	A low volume pulse which slowly rises and falls (plateau pulse) is seen in aortic stenosis.
Low volume	Other causes of a low volume pulse include mitral stenosis, pulmonary hypertension and shock.
High volume	A high volume pulse which rapidly rises then falls
Collapsing pulse	away abruptly (collapsing pulse) is seen particularly in aortic regurgitation but found also with high cardiac output states such as patent ductus arteriosus, pregnancy, a-v malformations, severe anaemia, hepatic cirrhosis, fever, thyrotoxicosis and also in complete heart block. It can be demonstrated at the wrist by placing the palm of the right hand over the radial artery and then elevating the patient's arm, keeping their elbow straight with your left hand. The pulse volume increases on elevation in patients with a collapsing pulse.
Jerky	A jerky upstroke is characteristic of hypertrophic obstructive cardiomyopathy. This condition can also
Bisferiens	produce the double beat (bisferiens) which is found more typically in combined aortic stenosis and regurgitation.
Dicrotic	An apparent second impulse with each beat (dicrotic) is felt in fever and hyperdynamic states.
Alternans	Alternating high and low volume beats (alternans) sometimes accompany left ventricular failure and may be confirmed using the sphygmomanometer.

Paradoxus

The volume of the pulse normally decreases slightly on inspiration but this is exaggerated (so called paradoxus) in cardiac tamponade, constrictive pericarditis and severe airways obstruction.

Inequality

Inequality between the radial pulses may be seen in Takayasu's disease and aortic aneurysm, whilst an absent radial pulse may suggest an embolus.

Absent radial

Radiofemoral delay

Delay in pulse transmission to the femoral arteries is found in coarctation of the aorta.

Blood pressure

The blood pressure, which must always be recorded in the cardiovascular examination, often confirms findings suspected from the character of the pulse. This recording may be left to the end of the examination.

Neck

Jugular venous pressure

The jugular venous pulse should then be inspected (see Ch. 5).

Precordium

Apex beat

The apex beat, the furthest downward and outward point at which the cardiac impulse is palpable, should be located. It is normally in the fifth intercostal space at the midclavicular line. Count down from the sternal angle which lies beside the second rib. The patient should be lying straight when the apex beat is examined.

Thrusting

A thrusting, heaving or sustained apex beat is found with left ventricular hypertrophy.

Tapping

A tapping apex beat, due to a palpable first heart sound, may be found in mitral stenosis.

Double impulse

A dyskinetic or aneurysmal segment of the left ventricle may lead to a double or diffuse impulse. A double impulse may also occur in hypertrophic obstructive cardiomyopathy.

Absent impulse

Dextrocardia

An absent apex beat may be due to pericardial effusion, obesity or emphysema; in dextrocardia the apex beat is found on the right side.

Pericardial knock

A pericardial 'knock' may occur in constrictive pericarditis.

Parasternal heave

A left parasternal heave should be sought and occurs in right ventricular hypertrophy. A palpable second heart sound occurs in pulmonary hypertension, whilst a pulsatile aortic arch aneurysm may be felt in the second right intercostal space.

Apical thrills	Apical thrills (palpable bruit) are systolic in mitral regurgitation and papillary muscle rupture and diastolic in mitral stenosis.
Parasternal thrill	A left parasternal thrill is associated with a ventricular septal defect.
Basal thrills	Thrills at the base of the heart again may be systolic in aortic or pulmonary stenosis or diastolic in aortic and pulmonary regurgitation. It is best to interpret thrills in combination with auscultatory findings.

Abdomen

Hepatomegaly	Hepatomegaly should be sought and has a smooth, rounded edge in congestive cardiac failure and may be pulsatile with tricuspid regurgitation.

PERCUSSION

Cardiac dullness	The area of cardiac dullness is variable and of limited value. However, increased right parasternal dullness may be detected in pericardial effusion and left atrial enlargement, whilst the absence of cardiac dullness occurs in obesity and emphysema.
Pleural effusions	Pleural effusions, detected by percussion over the base of the chest, may occur in cardiac failure (see Ch. 7).

AUSCULTATION

Auscultation of the heart (Fig. 6.1) should begin with the diaphragm of the stethoscope, listening in turn (1→8) at the apex, the axilla, the lower left parasternal area, the lower right parasternal area, the upper right parasternal area, the carotid arteries, the upper and mid left parasternal area (with the patient sitting forward in expiration) and finally with the bell at or just medial to the apex (with the patient turned on the left side and after exercise if necessary). Using this systematic approach, most sounds and murmurs will be identified.

Heart Sounds

First heart sound *Loud* *Soft*	The first heart sound is due mainly to mitral valve closure. It is loud in mitral stenosis and a hyperdynamic circulation, and soft in mitral regurgitation, calcified mitral stenosis, hypotension and severe heart failure. It varies in intensity in complete heart block and ventricular tachycardia.

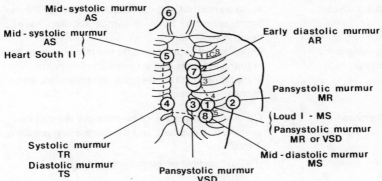

Fig. 6.1 Auscultation of the heart.

Split	The normal splitting of the first heart sound is more pronounced in right bundle branch block.
Second heart sound	The second heart sound is due to aortic and pulmonary valve closure and normally the aortic component occurs first in adults and is louder.
Split	Splitting of the second sound diminishes in expiration, whilst wide splitting occurs in pulmonary stenosis and left bundle branch block.
Fixed split	Fixed splitting (no change with respiration) occurs with atrial septal defect and right bundle branch block.
Reversed split	Paradoxical or reversed splitting (pulmonary before aortic component and decreasing on inspiration) may occur in left bundle branch block, severe aortic stenosis, left ventricular failure and patent ductus arteriosus.
Single	A single second sound may be heard in calcified aortic stenosis, pulmonary stenosis and common truncus arteriosus as well as appearing single in some normal elderly patients.
Third heart sound	The third heart sound is due to ventricular filling at the time of a-v valve opening and is normal in young people towards the cardiac apex. It also occurs where there is rapid ventricular filling—mitral regurgitation, ventricular septal defect, congestive cardiac failure and constrictive pericarditis.
Fourth heart sound	The fourth heart sound is due to ventricular filling as a result of atrial contraction and is heard in cardiac failure, myocardial infarction, hypertension and hypertrophic obstructive cardiomyopathy.

Gallop rhythm	A gallop rhythm, a tachycardia with added third or fourth sound (or both—summation gallop) may be heard in heart failure.
Opening snap *Ejection click*	Other added sounds include the opening snap heard in mitral stenosis and an ejection click heard sometimes in aortic stenosis, hypertension, and mitral valve prolapse.

Murmurs

Cardiac murmurs are conventionally divided into systolic and diastolic and the loudness graded from 1 to 6:

1—Just audible (in quiet surroundings)
2—Quiet
3—Moderately loud
4—Loud with palpable thrill
5—Very loud with pronounced thrill
6—Audible without the aid of stethoscope

As murmurs are sometimes graded from only 1—4 it is preferable always to indicate the scale used (e.g. 2/4 or 3/6). The characteristics of the commoner murmurs are listed in Table 6.1.

Systolic

Mid-systolic

Innocent	Innocent mid-systolic murmurs at the left sternal edge may be heard in hyperdynamic states, pregnancy and chest deformities.
Aortic stenosis	A mid-systolic murmur at the right upper sternal edge which radiates to the neck (and may radiate to the apex) is heard in aortic stenosis.
Aortic sclerosis	A similar murmur, sometimes with a mewing 'seagull's cry' quality is heard in aortic sclerosis.
Mitral valve prolapse *HOCM* *Pulmonary stenosis* *Atrial septal defect*	The mid-to-late systolic murmurs due to mitral valve prolapse or hypertrophic obstructive cardiomyopathy occur at the left sternal edge as do those of pulmonary stenosis and atrial septal defect.

Pansystolic

Mitral regurgitation *Ventricular septal defect*	Pansystolic murmurs at the apex due to mitral regurgitation radiate to the axilla whilst those due to ventricular septal defect radiate to the left sternal edge.
Ruptured chordae	Systolic murmurs associated with rupture of chordae tendinae may radiate to the right upper chest.

Table 6.1 Findings in common cardiac lesions.

Lesion	Murmur	Associated Signs
Aortic stenosis	Mid systolic at upper right sternal border (to neck/apex)	Thrill Click Faint aortic or single or reversed second sound Thrusting Apex Plateau Pulse BP—low systolic, small pulse pressure Pale complexion
Pulmonary stenosis	Mid systolic at upper left sternal border	Cyanosis RV heave Split second sound (soft P_2) JVP—large 'a' wave, small volume pulse
Aortic regurgitation	Blowing early diastolic at left sternal border	Thrusting displaced apex Head nodding Carotid pulsation Collapsing pulse BP—wide pulse pressure Femoral bruit
Mitral stenosis	Rumbling mid diastolic murmur at apex (plus pre-systolic except AF)	Palpable loud first sound Opening snap Mitral facies Peripheral cyanosis Small volume pulse, often AF
Mitral regurgitation	Pansystolic at apex (to axilla)	Thrusting displaced apex Thrill Third heart sound
VSD	Rough pansystolic at apex (to sternum)	No cyanosis (unless R→L shunt) Thrill Thrusting displaced apex
ASD	Pulmonary systolic	Fixed split second sound RV heave
PDA	Continuous machinery murmur at upper left of sternum (to back)	Thrusting apex BP—wide pulse pressure
Coarctation of aorta	Loud rough systolic at left lung apex, back and front	Scapular and internal mammary collaterals—bruits Radiofemoral delay Hypertension in arms

Tricuspid regurgitation	Tricuspid regurgitation murmurs occur at the right lower sternal edge especially on inspiration and are associated with hepatic pulsation and giant jugular venous 'v' waves.

Diastolic

Early diastolic

Aortic regurgitation	The early diastolic murmur of aortic regurgitation may be heard at any position down the left sternal edge and is accentuated by expiration, while
Pulmonary regurgitation	pulmonary regurgitation is accentuated by inspiration. An early diastolic murmur in the pulmonary area may be heard in pulmonary
Graham Steel	hypertension due to mitral stenosis (Graham Steel).

Mid Diastolic

Mitral stenosis	The mid-diastolic murmur of mitral stenosis is low-pitched and rumbling and heard at or just medial to the apex and may be accentuated by turning the patient on to the left side and by exercise (e.g. touching toes in bed).
Pre-systolic accentuation	A pre-systolic component to the murmur of mitral stenosis may be heard in sinus rhythm. An apical diastolic murmur is sometimes heard with aortic
Austin Flint	incompetence (Austin Flint).
Tricuspid stenosis	Tricuspid stenosis is rare and best heard at the right lower sternal edge.
Carey Coombs	A short diastolic murmur is heard with acute rheumatic mitral valvitis (Carey Coombs).

Continuous

	Continuous murmurs may be heard in coarctation of the aorta, arterio-venous shunts, patent ductus arteriosus and ruptured sinus of valsalva. A venous hum simulates a continuous murmur and may be abolished by light pressure on the side of the neck.
Posture	It should be remembered that change in posture can influence murmurs. For example, rising from the sitting position decreases venous return and therefore reduces the murmur of pulmonary and aortic stenosis, whilst increases the murmur associated with mitral valve prolapse and hypertrophic obstructive cardiomyopathy. Squatting increases cardiac afterload and increases aortic, pulmonary and mitral regurgitation.

Pericardial Rub

	A creaky, 'leathery' sound may be heard in

pericarditis, which may vary with respiration and posture. It may be systolic, diastolic or both. A pleuropericardial rub varies throughout the respiratory cycle.

Other Bruits

Carotid bruits should be sought and differentiated from cardiac murmurs. Femoral bruits are usually due to arthrosclerosis, but in aortic regurgitation a to-and-fro bruit may be produced by partially occluding the artery proximally (Duroziez's sign).

Lungs

Auscultation of the lung fields is essential, paying particular attention to the presence of crepitations and signs of chronic lung disease.

Blood Pressure

The blood pressure should be recorded in both the erect and supine position with a sphygmomanometer cuff of adequate size around the arm at the level of the heart (see also Ch. 17).

Fundi

The fundi should be examimed for changes particularly in hypertension and infective endocarditis (Roth spots).

7. RESPIRATORY SYSTEM

INSPECTION

Hands

It is conventional to start the examination of the respiratory system with the hands.

Finger clubbing

Finger clubbing (see Ch. 1) is an important clinical sign and occurs in association with certain pulmonary disorders, e.g. bronchiectasis, bronchial carcinoma, mesothelioma, asbestosis, empyema and fibrosing alveolitis.

Asterixis

A flapping tremor (asterixis) occurs in hypercapnia (Ch. 1). Other signs of CO_2 retention are dilated

Bounding pulse

veins, a bounding pulse, papilloedema, confusion and sweating.

Peripheral cyanosis

Peripheral cyanosis should be noted if present (see Ch. 12).

Face

Central cyanosis
Buccal mucosa

Central cyanosis (Ch. 12) is detected by inspecting the buccal mucosa and differentiates 'blue bloaters' from 'pink puffers' in chronic obstructive airways disease.

Moon face

A 'moon face' may be present and related to steroid therapy in obstructive airways disease.

Eyes

Horner's syndrome

Horner's syndrome (see Ch. 3) in a patient with chest disease is an important finding and usually indicates involvement of the cervical sympathetic nerves by an apical bronchial carcinoma (Pancoast's syndrome).

Chest and Neck

Accessory muscles of respiration

Use of the accessory muscles of respiration usually indicates respiratory difficulty. The patient frequently sits upright with arms extended supporting and fixing the chest thereby enabling these accessory muscles to help with respiration.

Chest Shape

Straight back	A straight or rigid back with decreased expansion is seen in ankylosing spondylosis.
Scoliosis	Scoliosis may be associated with rib or chest wall flattening and, if secondary to pulmonary disease, indicates a chronic disorder.
Kyphosis	Kyphosis may be severe enough (e.g. Pott's disease of spine) to impair respiration.
Barrel chest	Barrel deformity is an increase in anteroposterior diameter with thoracic kyphosis, ribs and clavicles more horizontal than usual, filling of supraclavicular fossa, and a subcostal angle greater than 90° and is often associated with emphysema.
Pectus carinatum	Pectus carinatum or pigeon chest is an increased prominence of upper sternum often due to rickets (look for Harrison's sulcus) or chronic chest infection.
Pectus excavatum	Pectus excavatum or funnel chest is a depression of lower sternum, is usually congenital and perhaps due to a short central diaphragmatic tendon.
Rickety rosary *Harrison's sulci*	Prominent costochondral epiphyses seen in rickets (rickety rosary), may be associated with Harrison's sulci, a deformity associated with indrawing of ribs below the nipple due to traction of diaphragm. This latter deformity may be seen in childhood asthma as well as rickets.
Intercostal drawing	Intercostal indrawing indicates increased negative intrathoracic pressure, usually associated with obstructive airways disease.
Expansion	Chest expansion is best inspected by observing the supine patient from the foot of the bed. Symmetry of expansion of both sides of chest should be checked.
Respiratory rate and pattern	The normal respiratory rate is approximately 14/min; an increased rate (tachypnoea) is seen in anxiety states, painful and restrictive chest diseases (where it is often shallow), pneumonia, pulmonary elbolism and left ventricular failure. Rapid and deep respiration is seen in states of metabolic acidosis such as diabetic ketoacidosis. Cheyne-Stokes respiration, cycles of increasing and decreasing depths of respiration, is seen in patients with

cerebral or respiratory depression associated with cerebrovascular disease, uraemia, cardiac failure and during sleep in the elderly.

PALPATION

Mediastinal displacement
Tracheal deviation

Mediastinal displacement is checked by assessing the position of the trachea and apex beat.
The tracheal position is the more important sign and should be checked in all patients. The neck should be slightly flexed and not rotated. Methods of assessing centrality include:
1) Insert the index and middle fingers into the suprasternal notch and feel for tracheal displacement *or*
2) Place the middle finger into the centre of the suprasternal notch with the second and fourth fingers on either side of the suprasternal notch feeling for the centre of the trachea *or*
3) Grip the trachea with the thumb and index finger and determine position.

Apex beat

The position of the apex beat should be noted, but it should be remembered that its position is influenced by heart size and displacement is only infrequently due to mediastinal displacement. The mediastinum is displaced to the left in collapse or fibrosis of left lower lobe, right pleural effusion or right pneumothorax and displaced to the right by left pneumothorax or pleural effusion, or fibrosis or collapse of the right lower lobe.

Crico-sternal distance

The distance between the cricoid cartilage and the sternal notch should be determined and is reduced in emphysema and during an asthmatic attack.

Lymphadenopathy (Supraclavicular & Axillary)

Supraclavicular (Ch. 5) and axillary lymphadenopathy should be noted.

Breasts

The breasts should be inspected for symmetry and nipple indrawing or discharge and skin changes. Examine with the patient's hands by her side, on her hips and held behind her head. Palpate with the palmar aspect of the fingers in a rotary fashion exerting initially gentle and later firmer pressure against chest wall. Examine each quadrant in turn.

Gynaecomastia

Gynaecomastia is the presence of increased breast tissue in men. It should be differentiated from obesity by the granular texture of periareolar tissue.

It may occur in liver disease, at puberty, in testicular teratomata and neoplasms such as carcinoma and lymphoma, in endocrine disorders such as hyperthyroidism, acromegaly and Addison's disease, Klinefelter's syndrome, renal failure and with drugs such as oestrogen, spironolactone, digoxin and cimetidine.

Chest expansion   Chest expansion should be measured as follows: the thumbs should be placed as vertical as is possible on either side of the midline with the fingers gripping firmly the patient's lateral chest wall; assess expansion anteriorly and posteriorly in upper and lower zones. Normal expansion should be at least 5 cm. Diminished expansion is seen with consolidation, atelectasis, lung abscess, fibrosis, pneumothorax and large pleural effusions.

Tactile vocal fremitus   Tactile vocal fremitus should be assessed with one hand on both sides of chest using the ulnar aspect of the cupped hand (or the palm) whilst the patient repeats the words '111' or '99'. Tactile vocal fremitus gives the same information as vocal resonance: increased in consolidation and reduced with pleural effusions and collapse.

PERCUSSION

Percussion of the chest should cover the upper, middle and lower segments — anteriorly, posteriorly and laterally. Two 'taps' are sufficient; the pleximeter finger should lie along or between, but not across, the ribs. Corresponding zones of the chest should be compared including the apices, which are assessed by percussing the clavicles directly. Anteriorly, dullness is usually found below the sixth rib and posteriorly, dullness is usually found at and below the tenth rib. These positions obviously vary with respiration.

Cardiac dullness   Loss of cardiac dullness is seen in emphysema, pneumothorax and obesity. Dextrocardia should be remembered as a cause of an apparent loss of cardiac dullness and the opposite side examined.

Hyperresonance Dullesss   Hyperresonance is a sign of over-inflation while dullness suggests consolidation, lung abscess, atelectasis and fibrosis. Stony dullness is detected over pleural effusions.

Percussion over the sternum may be used to confirm a retrosternal goitre.

Sternal tenderness	Percussion of the sternum may elicit tenderness due to marrow proliferation most commonly in acute leukaemia.

AUSCULTATION

Breath Sounds	The breath sounds over the upper, middle and lower zones anteriorly, posteriorly and laterally should be listened for using the diaphragm of the stethoscope.
Vesicular	Vesicular breath sounds demonstrate an inspiratory phase that is longer than the expiratory phase which follows without a pause; they are soft in character, compared with bronchial breath sounds,
Bronchial	which are longer and harsher with a prolonged expiratory phase which follows inspiration after a pause. Bronchial breath sounds are typically heard over consolidation but may also occur with fibrosis and above a pleural effusion.
Diminished	Breath sounds are diminished in atelectasis, fibrosis, pneumothorax and absent over a pleural effusion.

Added Sounds

Crepitations (crackles)	Crepitations are usually heard during inspiration. They are predominantly fine in early consolidation, medium in pulmonary oedema and coarse in bronchiectasis and fibrosing alveolitis. Crepitations which clear on coughing are not significant. Crepitations can also be classified by their timing, either as early or late inspiratory: the former due to airways obstruction and the latter in pulmonary oedema, fibrosing alveolitis and sarcoidosis.
Rhonchi (wheezes)	Rhonchi are musical blowing sounds which are usually heard in expiration; generalised expiratory rhonchi are characteristic of obstructive airways disease; localised rhonchi suggest focal structural disease. A silent chest in the face of a severe asthmatic attack has a grave prognosis without energetic treatment.
Pleural rub	Pleural rubs should be listened for. They are harsh creaking, usually localised sounds, associated with underlying pleural inflammation. Attendant pleuritic chest pain is frequently present.
Vocal resonance	Vocal resonance is elicited by asking the patient to repeat the words '111' and '99' whilst listening with the diaphragm of the stethoscope; corresponding

areas of each side of the chest should be compared. This provides similar information to tactile vocal fremitus; as before, increased in consolidation and reduced in pleural effusions and collapse.

Whispering pectoriloquy

Whispering pectoriloquy is elicited by asking the patient to whisper whilst listening with the diaphragm of the stethoscope; loud transmission of the sound is described as whispering pectoriloquy and may be heard above the fluid level of a pleural effusion and over pneumonic consolidation.

8. ABDOMEN

INSPECTION

Hands (see Ch. 1)

Finger clubbing

It is helpful to look briefly at the patient's hands and face before examining the abdomen. In particular, finger clubbing should be looked for and occurs in association with inflammatory bowel disease and hepatic cirrhosis (Ch. 1).

Leukonychia
Koilonychia
Palmar erythema
Dupuytren's contracture
Asterixis
Tylosis

Leukonychia occurs in hypoalbuminaemia and koilonychia in chronic iron deficiency.
Palmar erythema, Dupuytren's contracture and flapping tremor (asterixis) should be looked for specifically and, if present, should alert one to look for other stigmata of liver disease.
Tylosis of the palms is associated with carcinoma of the oesophagus.

Finger tip atrophy
Calcinosis

Atrophy of the finger tips with tightening of the overlying skin and calcinosis is seen in the CRST syndrome (**c**alcinosis, **R**aynaud's syndrome, **s**clerodactyly, **t**elangiectasia) and is associated with oesophageal motility disturbance.

Eyes

Jaundice
Conjunctival pallor
Kayser-Fleischer rings

The sclera should be inspected for jaundice and the conjunctiva for pallor of anaemia.
Kayser-Fleischer rings may be seen in hepato-lenticular degeneration (Wilson's disease) as brown rings at the outer corneal margin.

Xanthelasma

Xanthelasma may suggest primary biliary cirrhosis, especially in a jaundiced patient.

Face

Cachexia
Pallor
Sallow

A cachectic appearance may suggest an underlying malignancy, whilst pallor occurs in anaemia and a sallow complexion in renal failure.

Rhinophyma	Rhinophyma, a complication of acne rosacea, occurs with higher frequency in alcoholic patients.
Parotid swelling	Parotid enlargement may occur due to parotitis in alcoholic patients.

Mouth

Tongue *Furring*	The tongue should be inspected for furring which occurs in patients who breath through their mouths and is particularly seen in febrile patients and in liver failure and uraemia.
Glossitis	Glossitis may occur in iron deficiency anaemia which may complicate gastrointestinal bleeding and may be accompanied by angular cheilitis; it is also seen in the Paterson-Brown Kelly syndrome and in malabsorption states. A painful smooth tongue is seen in pernicious anaemia.
Jaundice	Yellow colouration of the frenulum of the tongue may occur early in hyperbilirubinaemia.
Aphthous ulcers	A small number of patients with aphthous ulceration of the tongue also have inflammatory bowel disease.
Angiomata	Angiomata of the tongue or lips should raise the possibility of hereditary haemorrhagic telangiectasia, especially in patients with gastrointestinal bleeding.
Foetor hepaticus	The sweet musty smell of foetor hepaticus and the distinctive odour of alcohol should be recognised.

Skin

	Many clues may be gained by a brief examination of the skin.
Scratch marks	Jaundice with scratch marks indicates cholestasis.
Pigmentation	Patients with primary biliary cirrhosis are yellow early in the disease but later develop a green-brown colour. Haemochromatosis (bronzed diabetes) is associated with a slatey-brown pigmentation.
Blisters	In porphyria cutanea tarda, which may be associated with alcoholic liver disease, the skin is fragile and blisters form with slight trauma and in sunlight. In females, this is associated with hirsutism.
Bruises	Bruises, in hospital patients, are frequently iatrogenic but do occur more often in alcoholics and patients with liver disease.
Tattooing	The association between tattooing and hepatitis B should be remembered.

Spider naevi (see Ch. 5)	Normal subjects seldom have more than six spider naevi and the presence of more should alert the examiner to chronic liver disease. An increased number of spider naevi is also seen during pregnancy (they disappear within a few months of delivery) and in rheumatoid arthritis. Spider naevi occur mainly in the region of drainage of the superior vena cava, and in particular on the anterior upper chest, neck, face and back of hands. They can be easily differentiated from Campbell de Morgan spots by their capacity to blanch on pressure.
Gynaecomastia	Gynaecomastia is associated with alcoholic cirrhosis and also with treatment of ascites with spironolactone (Ch. 7).
Dermatitis *Dermatitis herpetiformis*	Dermatitis may be associated with vitamin deficiency while dermatitis herpetiformis is associated with coeliac disease.
Pyoderma gangrenosum	Pyoderma gangrenosum may be seen in ulcerative colitis. A migratory necrolytic erythematous eruption may be seen with a glucagonoma.
Striae	Striae which may be red (if recent) or white, occur around the abdomen, shoulders, buttocks and thighs in pregnancy and obesity. In Cushing's syndrome, these striae tend to be purple in colour.
Abdomen	The abdomen should be inspected both from above and the side. The latter is most easily done by kneeling at the patient's bedside.
Shape	The shape of the abdomen may provide clues to underlying disease. A scaphoid abdomen occurs in starvation, malabsorption and wasting diseases. Abdominal distention, with evertion of the
Ascites	umbilicus, may be due to ascites, which occurs in decompensated cirrhosis, intra-abdominal malignancy, congestive cardiac failure, nephrotic syndrome, peritonitis, constrictive pericarditis, and the Budd-Chiari syndrome. Causes of distention, other than ascites (fluid) include intenstinal fluid, obesity (fat), gas (flatus), pregnancy (fetus) and faeces.
Scars	Scars should prompt questioning about previous surgical operations.
Veins	Dilated, tortuous veins occur in portal hypertension and vena caval obstruction. In portal hypertension,

veins tend to radiate from the umbilicus (caput medusa). In inferior vena caval obstruction, venous flow can be demonstrated to be in an upward direction both above and below the umbilicus whilst in superior vena caval obstruction, the flow is in the opposite direction.

Discolouration
Discolouration of the periumbilical area (Cullen's sign) or of the flank (Grey Turner's sign) may be noted with retroperitoneal haemorrhage and in particular in haemorrhagic pancreatitis.

Hernial orifices
Genitalia
The hernial orifices must always be inspected for herniae and lymphadenopathy. The genitalia must always be examined in clinical practice. Fistulae and fissures as well as haemorrhoids may be seen in the peri-anal area.

Pulsation
Abdominal pulsations are common in thin individuals but may suggest the presence of an aortic aneurysm. Small intestinal peristalsis may also be seen in thin individuals but will be unduly prominent in intestinal obstruction and their position may give an indication as to the site of obstruction.

Abdominal wall
movement
Diminished movement of the abdominal wall muscles is seen in peritonitis.

PALPATION

General

Tenderness
After asking the patient to indicate areas of tenderness, which should be examined last, palpation should start lightly, assessing muscle tone and outlining superficial masses. Areas of tenderness should be examined gently, testing for guarding (voluntary muscular contraction) and rebound tenderness. The presence of the latter implies inflammation of the parietal peritoneum. The patient's face must be watched for signs of pain.

Masses
The abdomen should then be palpated more deeply to identify intra-abdominal masses. The size, shape, consistency, tenderness, mobility, attachment, fluctuation and associated lymphadenopathy of any mass should be recorded.

Specific

Specific examination for enlargement of the liver, spleen, kidneys and bladder should be carried out systematically in the supine patient.

Liver

Two main methods of palpating the liver exist. In the most common method, the palpating (right) hand is placed with the index finger lying parallel with the costal margin. Alternatively, the fingers of one or both hands are placed at 90° to the costal margin. In both methods, the liver is felt descending on deep inspiration as controlled firm pressure is applied. The edge is felt with the side of the index finger in the first method and the tips of the fingers using the second. The liver border is palpable in the epigastrium and just below the right costal margin on deep inspiration in normal subjects. Care should be taken not to miss the lower border of a massively enlarged liver in the right iliac fossa.

Upper border

Not all livers that are easily palpable are enlarged and the upper border must be determined by percussion to enable the apparently large liver to be differentiated from the displaced low-lying liver in emphysema.

Riedel's lobe

A Riedel's lobe, an anatomical variant of the right lobe commoner in females, must be distinguished from hepatomegaly and the right kidney.

Hepatomegaly

The commonest causes of hepatomegaly in the UK are cirrhosis, carcinoma and congestive cardiac failure (the 3 C's). Other common causes include fatty liver, myeloproliferative disease and hepatitis (Table 8.1).

Spleen

The spleen is a relatively superficial organ and will be missed by too-deep palpation. Examination is bimanual with the left hand placed postero-laterally over the lower left costal margin with the right hand flat on the abdomen with the fingers pointing towards the left hand. The edge of the spleen descends from under the costal margin in deep inspiration and meets the fingers of the right hand. Examination should begin in the right iliac fossa. The spleen is not felt in health and is only palpable once it has enlarged to 3−4 times its normal size. In situations where the spleen is only just palpable, rolling the patient on to their right side may allow it to be more easily felt. The spleen should be distinguished from the left kidney by five characteristics:

1) It moves freely with respiration
2) You cannot get above the swelling

Table 8.1 Causes of hepatomegaly in UK.

Common	Uncommon
Cardiac failure (congestion)	Malaria
Carcinoma (metastases, hepatoma, lymphoma)	Polycystic liver
Cirrhosis	Riedel's lobe
Myeloproliferative disease	Storage diseases (amyloidosis, Gaucher's, Niemann-Pick and glycogen-storage diseases)
Viral hepatitis	Budd-Chiari syndrome
Fatty liver	Non-viral infections (TB, hydatid cyst, amoebic abscess, Weil's disease, toxoplasmosis,
Biliary obstruction	schistosomiasis)

3) It has a notch on its medial border
4) Overlying dullness to percussion
5) A space exists between its posterior edge and erector spinae muscles.

Not all these characteristics are present in all patients.

Splenomegaly The commonest causes of an enlarged spleen in the UK are shown in Table 8.2

Kidneys The kidneys are frequently not palpable in health, although the lower border of the right kidney may be felt easily in thin patients. Palpation should be bimanual with the left hand posteriorly below the 12th rib and the right hand anteriorly. At the end of deep inspiration, the posterior hand should ballot the kidney onto the deeply palpating right hand. The

Table 8.2 Causes of splenomegaly in UK.

Massive	Large	Just Palpable
Chronic myeloid leukaemia	Portal hypertension	Infective endocarditis
Myelofibrosis	Polycythaemia rubra vera	Infectious mononucleosis
	Chronic lymphatic leukaemia	
	Lymphoma	
	Haemolytic anaemias	
	Storage disease	

normal kidney has a characteristic firm and smooth surface.

Renal enlargement See Chapter 14.

Adrenal Adrenal masses may be palpable and enlarge posteriorly, obliterating the angle between the 12th rib and supra-spinatus muscle.

Bladder The bladder is felt arising from the pelvis usually in the midline. In the female, it should be differentiated from the pregnant uterus, uterine fibroids and ovarian cysts.

Other masses After carefully palpating the abdomen for the above organs, the rest of the abdomen should be systematically palpated. A palpable gallbladder may be noted in the right hypochondrium while an epigastric mass may indicate a gastric carcinoma. The caecum and rectosigmoid colon are often palpable in thin patients; masses in the colon may be neoplastic but should be tested to see if they are indentable (faeces). Uterine and ovarian masses may also be identified.

Fluid thrill Where it is indicated (i.e. in patients with abdominal distention) a fluid thrill, if present, should be elicited. A dividing hand over the centre of the abdomen is unnecessary in non-obese patients.

Ballottment/dipping When a large volume of ascitic fluid is present, 'dipping' or ballottment may be the only way to identify organomegaly or masses. This is done by rapid depression of the fingertips which, by displacement of fluid, produces a tapping sensation over organs beneath.

Succussion splash Rocking the patient from side-to-side may produce a succussion splash due to fluid in the stomach. It is only abnormal (indicating gastric stasis or outlet obstruction) if still present 2 − 3 hours post prandially.

Pulses *Hernial orifices* The femoral pulses should routinely be palpated at the same time as palpating the hernial orifices. An inguinal hernia originates above the pubic tubercle and may be indirect or direct. A femoral hernia lies in the femoral canal below and lateral to the pubic tubercle. Umbilical, epigastric and incisional hernias may also be noted. All hernias should be examined, their contents identified and their reducibility assessed. A non-reducible hernia which is tender should suggest strangulation.

Rectal Examination

The rectal examination is important in clinical practice and should be performed in all patients. The procedure should first be explained and the patient put on their left side with knees drawn up to the chest. Adequate lubricating jelly on the gloved finger must be used. The anus should be entered slowly and its tone assessed.

Prostrate

In males, the prostate should be palpated and the median sulcus identified. The texture and size of the gland should be assessed.

Cervix

In the female, the cervix and the lateral fornices should be palpated.

The remaining three quadrants of the anal canal should be examined in turn, feeling for ulceration, polyps, masses and tenderness.

Masses

Remember that piles, unless thrombosed or very large, are seldom palpable. After the finger is withdrawn, the glove should be inspected for blood and faecal occult blood tested for, if indicated.

PERCUSSION

Percussion should be used to confirm both upper and lower borders of the liver and to confirm enlargement of the spleen, as these organs are examined. The upper border of the liver usually lies at the level of the sixth rib anteriorly. The lower border of the liver should be percussed gently, and always from the area of resonance to the area of dullness.

Shifting dullness

Percussion is also used to confirm the presence of ascites by eliciting shifting dullness. Once dullness in both flanks has been identified in the supine patient, the line of transition from resonance to dullness should be noted and the patient rolled towards that side whilst keeping the left hand on the line of transition. If fluid is present, the area of dullness will have advanced towards the midline.

Puddle sign

The puddle sign of periumbilical dullness to percussion with the patient 'on all fours' can be used to identify small volumes of ascites but is seldom used in clinical practice.

Bladder size

Bladder size can be estimated by percussion.

AUSCULTATION

During the above examination, borborygmi, if audible, should be noted and may indicate intestinal obstruction. They are however, common in normal subjects.

Bowel Sounds	The normal frequency of bowel sounds varies considerably, although more than 30 per minute is usually abnormal and, particularly if loud, suggestive of early intestinal obstruction. Auscultation for at least 30 seconds is necessary before bowel sounds can be declared 'absent'. Diminished or absent bowel sounds occur in peritonitis. In late intestinal obstruction and paralytic ileus, the bowel sounds are high pitched and 'tinkling'.
Vascular bruit	Vascular bruits should be listened for specifically, although not all bruits are pathological, especially in the young.
Vessel-stenosis	Bruits may arise from stenosis of any intra-abdominal artery, although the site of maximal intensity will help to localise which vessel is involved.
Hepatic bruit	Hepatic bruits occur in hepatocellular carcinoma, alcoholic hepatitis and metastatic lesions. Rarely a splenic bruit is heard over an enlarged spleen.
Venous hum	A loud venous hum at the umbilicus associated with abdominal wall venous dilatation make up the Cruveilhier-Baumgarten syndrome, usually due to cirrhosis with a congenitally patent umbilical vein. Such a murmur is diagnostically useful in that it implies portal vein patency as the umbilical vein drains into the portal vein.
Perisplenic rub	A rub (analagous to pleural rub) may be heard over an area of splenic infarction.

9. LEGS

INSPECTION The skin of the lower limbs should be inspected.

Atrophy Atrophy of the skin is associated with peripheral
Loss of hair vascular disease, together with loss of hair, loss of
Pallor sweating and pale, cold extremeties.
Gangrene Cyanosis or gangrene may be seen. Peripheral
vascular disease is accelerated in diabetes mellitus
when sensory changes may also be present (see
Ulceration Ch. 15). These changes together with infection lead
to ulceration, which frequently affect pressure
points.

Athlete's foot Tinea infection of the feet (athlete's foot), seen as
flaky lesions between the toes, is common;
persistent or extensive infection may be associated
with peripheral vascular disease.

Raynaud's Raynaud's phenomenon causes white, cold,
phenomenon insensitive peripheries followed by cyanosis and
then redness. If severe, atrophic changes may occur
with time. Causes include connective tissue
diseases, cryoglobulinaemia, drugs (ergotamine)
and idiopathic.

Oedema Ankle oedema should be looked for specifically. If
present, a check should be made to see if pitting on
pressure occurs. The pressure must be applied for at
least five seconds over a bony landmark, usually the
lower tibia. Pitting oedema is usually due to
congestive cardiac failure, hypoalbuminaemia or
venous insufficiency.

Lymphoedema Painless swelling of the legs occurs in lymphoedema
which affects mainly the dorsal aspect of the feet
and toes, is brawny in colour and pits poorly on
pressure. It can occur in Milroy's disease, neoplasia
and elephantiasis.

Varicose veins *Stasis dermatitis*	Varicose veins may be seen together with stasis dermatitis or ulceration above and behind the medial malleoli.
Ulceration	Ulceration of the legs also may be associated with peripheral vascular disease, diabetes, neuropathy (e.g. due to alcohol, tabes, syringomyelia), infection, haemolytic anaemia, connective tissue diseases, trauma and neoplasia.
Deep vein thrombosis *Baker's cyst*	Swelling of the leg with oedema, redness or duskiness and dilated superficial veins may be seen in deep venous thrombosis; a ruptured Baker's cyst can cause similar changes in the calf.
Necrobiosis lipoidica	The raised red lesions with necrotic centres of necrobiosis lipoidica may be seen in diabetes.
Pretibial myxoedema	The mauve coloured pretibial swelling of pretibial myxoedema may be seen in hyperthyroidism.
Erythema nodosum	Raised erythematous discrete nodules of erythema nodosum may be seen with drug sensitivity (penicillin, sulphonamides), streptococcal and mycoplasmal infections, tuberculosis, leprosy, sarcoidosis, rheumatoid arthritis, rheumatic fever, ulcerative colitis and systemic fungal infections.
Vasculitis	Palpable purpuric spots with necrotic centres may be seen with vasculitis in connective tissue diseases and meningococcal septicaemia.
Purpura *Ecchymoses*	Purpura may first be noted in the legs and occurs when platelet defects are present, whilst ecchymoses suggest a coagulopathy or endothelial fragility (e.g. scurvy).
Keratoderma blenorrhagica	See Chapter 19.
Toe clubbing	Clubbing of the toes may occur in some patients with finger clubbing and carries the same significance.
Muscle wasting	The musculature should be inspected for wasting. This is generalised in cachexia, but proximal in osteomalacia, limb-girdle dystrophy, thyroid disease, Cushing's syndrome, and diabetic amytrophy. Distal wasting is seen in peripheral neuropathies such as peroneal muscle atrophy, whilst localised muscle wasting is typical of peripheral nerve lesions. Wasting and deformity of one leg may suggest old poliomyelitis.
Length	If one leg appears to be shortened, the true length of each leg should be measured from the anterior

superior iliac spine to the medial malleolus. Apparent shortening, due to pelvic tilt, will then become obvious.

Foot drop — Drop foot may be due to lateral popliteal nerve damage, prolapsed intervertebral disc, polyneuropathy or simply prolonged bed-rest.

Fasciculation — Fasciculation may be noted in lower motor neurone lesions as occurs in amyotrophic lateral sclerosis, cervical spondylosis, syringomyelia and root compression due to prolapse of a lumbar intervertebral disc.

Abnormal movements/posture — Inspect for abnormal movements — athetosis, tremor or spasm, and postural abnormalities (e.g. pes cavus, genu valgus or varus, and internal or external rotation).

PALPATION

Arterial pulses — The main arterial pulses in the legs should be checked (i.e. femoral, popliteal, posterior tibial and dorsalis pedis).

Temperature — Cold peripheries occur with both arterial and venous insufficiency. Deep venous thrombosis is associated with an increased temperature in the affected leg which is usually also tender. The leg circumference should be measured if one leg appears swollen or wasted.

Superficial thrombophlebitis — The tender, warm, red, palpable thrombosed veins of superficial thrombophlebitis should be noted if present.

Varicose veins — Varicose veins can be tested by Trendelenberg test i.e. elevate the leg then apply pressure over the origin of the long saphenous vein. If the patient then stands up and the veins do not fill, the long saphenous vein is competent.

Joints — Examination of joints is outlined in Chapter 19.

Tone — Tone should be assessed in a relaxed patient. Rolling the leg back and forth on the bed may give some idea of tone. However, the hip, knee and ankle should be put through a full range of passive movements for tone to be fully assessed.

Hypotonia — Hypotonia occurs in lower motor neurone lesions and acute upper motor neurone lesions, whilst

Spasticity — hypertonia with spasticity (clasp knife) is seen in established upper motor neurone lesions.

Plastic rigidity *'Cog-wheeling'*	Plastic (lead-pipe) rigidity occurs in Parkinsonism with 'cog-wheeling' when a superimposed tremor is present.
Power	Power should be tested in the muscle groups shown in Table 9.1. In lower motor neurone lesions diminished power is associated with flaccid wasted muscles and fasciculation, whilst in upper motor neurone lesions diminished power coexists with increased tone, minor muscle wasting and clonus.
Coordination	See Chapter 18.
Gait	Certain typical gait patterns are described in Table 9.2.
Reflexes	The knee (L3,4) and ankle jerks (L5,S1) should be elicited and clonus looked for if hyperreflexia is present.
Hyporeflexia	Hyporeflexia occurs in lower motor neurone lesions, myopathies and with acute upper motor neurone damage.
Absent jerks	Retest with reinforcement before saying reflexes are absent.
Hyperreflexia	Hyperreflexia occurs in upper motor neurone lesions, thyrotoxicosis, hepatic coma and uraemia.
Pendular jerks	Pendular reflex jerks occur with cerebellar lesions, whilst a slow relaxation phase is typical in hypothyroidism.
Plantar reflex	The plantar reflex (L5,S1) elicited by stroking the lateral border of the sole of the foot, is flexor in normal subjects and extensor (Babinski's sign) in upper motor neurone lesions.
Oppenheim's test	Oppenheim's test is an equivalent test and is elicited by applying pressure along the anterior surface of the tibia.
Rossolimo's sign	Rossolimo's sign, elicited by flicking the distal phalanges of the toes in an extensor direction, produces brisk plantar flexion of the great toe in upper motor neurone lesions. Absent knee and ankle jerks, associated with an extensor plantar reflex, is seen in tabes dorsalis, subacute combined degeneration of cord, diabetic neuropathy, motor neurone disease and Friedreich's ataxia.

Table 9.1   Muscle group for power testing.

Group	Roots
Hip flexion	L1,2,3 (iliopsoas)
Hip extension	L5 (glutei)
Knee extension	L3,4 (quadriceps)
Knee flexion	L5,S1 (hamstrings)
Ankle dorsiflexion	L4,5
Ankle plantar flexion	S1,2 (gastrocnemius)
Ankle inversion	L4 (ant. & post. tibial)
Ankle eversion	L5,S1 (peronei)
Toe extension	L5,S1
Toe flexion	S2,3

Table 9.2   Some typical gait patterns.

Gait	Pattern	Cause
Hemiplegic	Extended leg, flexed arm Pelvis tilts to allow affected leg round and forward	Cerebrovascular accident

Paraparetic
  (Scissor)
	Stiffness of both legs
	Feet remain on ground
		Cerebral palsy, cord
		  compression, multiple
		  sclerosis, syringomyelia

Cerebellar	Wide-based, reeling,
	  unsteady, staggering
	  towards lesion
		Cerebellar lesions, multiple
		  sclerosis, alcoholism,
		  myxoedema

Festinating	Rigidity, shuffling, festination with stooped posture	Parkinson's disease

Waddling	Hips tilted alternately
	  (glutei weak)
		Congenital dislocation of the
		  hips
		Proximal myopathy
		Limb-girdle dystrophy
		Old polio

Steppage	Foot drop, high lift, slaps on
	  floor
		Lateral popliteal nerve palsy,
		  Peroneal muscular atrophy

Stamping	High stepping, wise base,
	  stamps (loss of position
	  sense)
		B_{12} deficiency, tabes dorsalis,
		  diabetes mellitus

Marche à petit pas	Small steps taken Stooped posture	Elderly, Parkinsonism
Astasia-abasia	Small steps Tendency to fall backwards	Elderly, Parkinsonism

Other Signs

Kernig's sign

Kernig's sign, elicited by flexing the hip and knee followed by knee extension, produces hamstring spasm in meningism.

Straight leg raising test

A prolapsed intervertebral disc at L5/S1 produces pain in the back of the leg if the hip is flexed with the knee extended (the straight leg raising test).

Femoral nerve stretch test

Prolapse of the intervertebral disc at L2/3 produces pain in the back if the knee is flexed in a prone patient with extended hips (the femoral nerve stretch test).

Sensation

Light touch
Pin prick
Temperature

Check sensation using both light touch and pin prick. Temperature sensation should only be tested in certain patients. Remember the dermatomes: L1—inguinal area; L2,3—anterior thigh; L4,5—shin, S1—lateral border foot, sole, back of calf.

Vibration

Vibration should be tested with a low frequency (128 Hz) tuning fork on the malleoli, patellae and anterior superior iliac spines. Position sense should be tested by either wiggling the toes, initially very gently with a gradually increasing arc and asking when the movement is felt, or by the conventional method of asking the patient to identify upward and downward movements. Loss of sensation is symmetrical and distal in neuropathy due to diabetes mellitus, thiamine deficiency, carcinomatous neuropathy and drugs. Dorsal column damage produces vibration sense loss (without spinothalamic loss) in both legs in vitamin B_{12} deficiency and tabes dorsalis and in the ipsilateral leg in the Brown-Sequard syndrome (where the contralateral leg has spinothalamic loss).

Sensory inattention

The inability to discriminate the fact that both legs are being touched at once while each leg is correctly identified when touched separately is sensory inattention and is seen with parietal lobe lesions particularly of the non-dominant cerebral hemisphere.

10. ANAEMIA

Not all pale looking patients are anaemic, whilst severe anaemia may be missed clinically unless looked for. As well as identifying the presence of anaemia, examination may provide important clues as to its aetiology and effects.

INSPECTION

General

Pallor

Generalised pallor may suggest anaemia, but other causes of pallor such as shock and panhypopituitarism should be borne in mind.

Palmar creases
Mucous membranes

Pallor of skin creases of the hands should be present as well as pallor of the mucous membranes (mouth, conjunctivae) before concluding that a patient is anaemic.

Cachexia

The cause of anaemia may be suggested from the general appearance—the cachexia of cancer, the archetypal white hair, blue eyes and lemon tinge to the skin of pernicious anaemia, and pregnancy (folate and iron deficiency).

Pernicious anaemia
Pregnancy
Racial origin

The racial origin of the patient should be noted. Haemoglobinopathies are commoner in Negroes and Asiatics, while thalassaemia is commoner around the Mediterranean coast and the Far East.

Stature

Shortness of stature occurs with the hereditary anaemias.

Oedema

Ankle oedema should be looked for and may indicate right heart failure secondary to anaemia.

Skin

Apart from pallor, characteristic changes occur in certain specific anaemias.

Jaundice

Jaundice occurs in haemolytic anaemias, neoplastic invasion of the liver, and chronic liver disease, whilst

Uraemia

in uraemia a muddy complexion is characteristic.

Hypothyroidism	The features of hypothyroidism are described in Chapter 2.
Ecchymoses	Ecchymoses may be present suggesting a coagulopathy or scurvy. In the latter there may be perifollicular haemorrhages.
Petechiae	Petechiae suggest a platelet-production problem such as auto-immune thrombocytopemia aplastic anaemia, leukaemia, lymphoma or secondary replacement of the marrow with cancer. The Hess test, where a sphygmomanometer cuff is inflated to the mid-way point between systolic and diastolic pressures for 5 minutes, may disclose a petechial tendency.
Dermatitis	An exfoliative dermatitis may mean an underlying lymphoma.
Psoriasis	Severe psoriasis may be treated with methotrexate causing a secondary folate-deficiency anaemia.
Scars	Scars of abdominal surgery may suggest 'post-gastrectomy' as a cause of anaemia.

Nails

Brittleness *Koilonychia*	Iron deficiency causes brittle nails and koilonychia, a characteristic spoon-shaped deformity.
Clubbing	Clubbing of the nails may be associated with anaemia in malabsorption states, ulcerative colitis, carcinoma or infective endocarditis.
Splinter haemorrhages	Infective endocarditis may also give rise to splinter haemorrhages.
Lindsay's nails	Chronic renal failure may be associated with Lindsay's nails — pallor of the nails with a distal brown arc.

Hands

Rheumatoid arthritis *Osteoarthrosis*	Examination of the hands may reveal typical changes of rheumatoid arthritis or osteoarthrosis. In the former, the primary disease state may contribute to the anaemia, while in both diseases, the treatment may cause anaemia (e.g. anti-inflammatory drugs causing gastrointestinal blood loss).
Dactylitis	Dactylitis, seen as a swollen and often tender finger, occurs in some haemoglobinopathies, especially sickle-cell disease as well as syphilis, sarcoidosis and tuberculosis.

Eyes

Conjunctival pallor should be looked for as should icterus. Conjunctival haemorrhages may be seen in leukaemia. Fundal changes which may occur are mentioned in Chapter 3.

Mouth/Tongue

Glossitis

Atrophic glossitis, a smooth, red and often painful tongue, occurs in iron, vitamin B12 and folic acid deficiency anaemias.

Mucous Membranes

Pallor is common to all anaemias.

Telangiectases

Small telangiectases may be seen in the mouth as well as on the skin in hereditary haemorrhagic telangiectasia.

Cheilitis

Cracking and soreness of the angle of the lips, angular cheilitis, is seen in iron and B vitamin deficiencies and with ill-fitting dentures.

Gums

Hypertrophy

Hypertrophy of the gums is seen with chronic phenytoin use which may cause folate deficiency. Hypertrophy with bleeding and infection is seen in the rare acute monocytic leukaemia.

Blue lines

Blue lines occur in lead poisoning which causes haemolytic anaemia and is a marrow toxin.

Bleeding

Bleeding from the gums is seen in scurvy and in thrombocytopenia but only if the patient has teeth. The association of swollen bleeding gums with

Vincent's angina

halitosis should suggest Vincent's angina.

Pharynx

Ulceration of the pharynx and tonsillar swelling may be seen in leukaemia, lymphoma or aplastic anaemia.

PALPATION

Pulse

The pulse rate and volume should be recorded and may provide information regarding the severity of the anaemia.

Lymphadenopathy

Localised lymphadenopathy may accompany a primary neoplasm such as Troissier's sign (left supraclavicular (Virchow's) node swelling in gastric carcinoma), while generalised lymphadenopathy would favour lymphoma or chronic lymphatic leukaemia. The lymph nodes involved by lymphoma are frequently rubbery in nature in distinction to the hard craggy nodes of metastatic carcinoma.

Abdomen	Tenderness in the epigastrium may occur in peptic ulcer disease.
Hepatomegaly	Hepatomegaly can occur in alcohol-related chronic liver disease which is also associated with poor diet, iron metabolism problems, folate deficiency or gastric bleeding. It may also occur in congestive cardiac failure secondary to anaemia.
Splenomegaly	Splenomegaly is massive in chronic myeloid leukaemia and myelofibrosis; moderate or just palpable in lymphomas, portal hypertension, haemolytic anaemias (except sickle-cell) and pernicious anaemia.
Kidneys	Large polycystic kidneys may be palpable and be responsible for renal failure.
Masses	A palpable mass may suggest an underlying malignancy of the stomach or colon.
Rectal	Rectal examination may reveal melaena, faeces positive for faecal occult blood, haemorrhoids or tumour.
Pelvis	Pelvic examination may reveal the cause of menorrhagia.

CNS

Subacute combined degeneration	Subacute combined degeneration of the cord may accompany pernicious anaemia and is identified by loss of vibration and position sense of the lower limbs, together with a 'glove-and-stocking' sensory loss. Ankle and knee jerks may also be lost. Lead poisoning may cause a distal motor neuropathy.
Meningism	Meningism may be seen in acute leukaemias with CNS involvement.

PERCUSSION

Percussion is of limited use in assessing a patient with anaemia other than in detecting sternal or vertebral tenderness in neoplastic disease.

AUSCULTATION

Heart murmurs	Auscultation of the heart may reveal 'flow' murmurs which resolve once the anaemia is treated. Heart murmurs associated with anaemia occur in infective endocarditis. The blood pressure should always be
Blood pressure	recorded and frequently shows a wide pulse pressure in anaemic patients. The presence of a postural drop in particular should raise the possibility of an actively bleeding lesion.

Table 10.1 Physical signs in common anaemias.

Iron deficiency	B12 deficiency	Underlying neoplasm
Pallor	Pallor	Pallor
CVS signs	CVS signs	CVS signs
Koilonychia	Jaundice	Palpable tumour
Glossitis	Premature greying	Cachexia
Angular cheilitis	Glossitis, glossodynia	Clubbing
	Subacute combined degeneration of the cord	Lymphadenopathy
		Often also signs of iron deficiency

11. POLYCYTHAEMIA

Examination of patients with polycythaemia may indicate the cause and may also show complications of the condition. Polycythaemia is defined as a raised red cell mass ($>6 \times 10^6$ RBC/ml or haematocrit >0.55) and is due to increased production of red cells. This may be primarily due to increased marrow production (polycythaemia rubra vera) or secondary to hypoxia—high altitude, haemoglobinopathies, cyanotic congenital heart disease, chronic obstructive airways disease, renal disease (cysts and tumours), uterine fibroids, hepatoma and cerebellar haemangioblastoma. Spurious polycythaemia (due to relative high red cell mass with a low plasma volume) is associated with smoking, anxiety and hypertension.

INSPECTION
General

Plethora	Facial plethora is often noted in polycythaemia, often with cyanosis (due to desaturation of more than 5 g/l haemoglobin).
Conjunctival injection	Conjunctival injection may also be present. Central cyanosis is often seen in cyanotic congenital heart disease and chronic obstructive airways disease.
Nicotine staining	Nicotine staining of fingers is common in smokers, who may have chronic obstructive airways disease or spurious polycythaemia (due to decreased plasma volume).
Clubbing	Clubbing of fingernails may be seen in cyanotic congenital heart disease and bronchial carcinoma.
Gout	Gouty tophi and hot, tender, swollen, red joints may be seen in gout which may complicate primary polycythaemia.

Obesity	Marked obesity associated with somnolence may give rise to secondary polycythaemia in the Pickwickian syndrome, due to hypoventilation.
Chest	Tachynpnoea and dyspnoea may be noted in patients with chronic obstructive airways disease who will also have diminished chest expansion. Cyanotic congenital heart disease may have other clinical signs (see Ch. 6).

Legs

PVD	Signs of peripheral vascular disease—white, cold legs with diminished sweating, atrophic skin with loss of hair and perhaps ulceration and gangrene— may be noted and are due to the hyperviscosity associated with polycythaemia.
DVT	Polycythaemia also predisposes to deep venous thrombosis (hot, swollen, tender calf with bluish discolouration and distended superficial veins).

PALPATION

Abdomen

Hepatosplenomegaly	Hepatosplenomegaly is often found in primary polycythaemia while hepatomegaly alone may be due to hepatoma.
Large kidneys	Large kidneys may be due to hydronephrosis, renal cysts, polycystic disease and renal adenocarcinoma (hypernephroma).
Uterine fibroids	Giant uterine fibroids may cause polycythaemia.
Rectal examination	Faeces positive for occult blood obtained at rectal examination may reflect the higher incidence of gastrointestinal haemorrhage in polycythaemia.

CNS

Cerebellar signs	Examination of the CNS may reveal cerebellar signs associated with cerebellar haemangioblastoma— ipsilateral ataxia, incoordination, nystagmus, hypotonia, pendular tendon jerks, pass-pointing, dysdiadochokinesis (see Ch. 18). It may also reveal
CVA	signs of a cerebrovascular accident (hemiplegia with increased tone, hyperreflexia and hemianopia) which may complicate polycythaemia.
Fundal examination	Engorged retinal veins with a dark background may be seen.

PERCUSSION

Percussion may be used to demonstrate hyperresonance in an emphysematous chest and is useful in confirming organomegaly on abdominal examination.

AUSCULTATION

Bruit

Arterial bruit may be present in patients with peripheral vascular disease. A bruit may also be heard over a hepatoma.

Blood pressure

The blood pressure should be checked since spurious polycythaemia may be associated with hypertension and anxiety. Hypertension is however also commoner in primary polycythaemia.

12. CYANOSIS

Patients with suspected cyanosis must be examined in good, natural light. The blue discolouration of cyanosis is due to an excess of reduced haemoglobin in the capillaries. Over 5 g/dl of haemoglobin must be present before cyanosis is apparent (i.e. approximately less than 85% saturated or PaO_2 less than 60 mmHg). Cyanosis must be classified as peripheral or central.

Peripheral Cyanosis

Peripheral cyanosis is due to low cardiac output, peripheral vascular disease, increased tissue oxygen extraction and extreme cold weather.

Central Cyanosis

Central cyanosis is due to inadequate oxygenation of the blood; causes include acute and chronic lung disease, pulmonary embolism, hypoventilation, decrease in inspired oxygen, polycythaemia, and right-to-left cardiac shunts.

Differential Cyanosis

Differential cyanosis with normal upper limbs and cyanosed lower limbs occurs with reversal of the shunt across a patent ductus arteriosus.

INSPECTION

Face

Buccal mucosa/ tongue
Lips

In central cyanosis there is always cyanosis at the periphery but the distinguishing feature is cyanosis of the buccal mucosa, tongue and lips.

Hands

In peripheral cyanosis the hands are cold and blue, as are other exposed parts.

Clubbing

Clubbing of the fingers is seen in cyanotic congenital heart disease and fibrotic lung disease (Ch. 1).

Flapping tremor

A flapping tremor in an acute exacerbation of

chronic bronchitis or emphysema reflects carbon dioxide retention (Ch. 1), while a fine tremor may reflect the use of sympathomimetic bronchodilators in these conditions.

Legs

Venous stasis

Ankle oedema

DVT

Poor venous drainage with stasis results in cyanosis and can be assessed by the time it takes for veins to empty on elevating the leg; ankle oedema is frequently found in this condition

Signs of deep venous thrombosis may or may not be seen in association with a pulmonary embolus.

Neck

Elevated JVP

Accessory muscles

Trachea

The jugular venous pressure may be elevated in cor pulmonale, pulmonary hypertension or pulmonary embolism.

Accessory muscles of respiration are frequently used in chronic bronchitis and emphysema.

Shortening of the crico-sternal distance (Ch. 7) occurs in obstructive airways disease.

Chest

Dyspnoea
Tachypnoea

Barrel chest
Pigeon chest

Hypoventilation with a slow respiratory rate may cause central cyanosis and occurs with cerebrovascular accidents and with drug overdosage.

Dyspnoea with a fast respiratory rate may occur in acute exacerbations of chronic bronchitis and emphysema, pulmonary embolism and sometimes in cyanotic congenital heart disease.

Barrel chest deformity is associated with chronic bronchitis and emphysema while a pigeon chest is sometimes seen in cyanotic congenital heart disease.

PALPATION

Pulse

Peripheral pulses

Tachycardia

Peripheral pulses may be weak or absent in peripheral vascular disease and should be checked.

A tachycardia may be associated with bronchodilator use and occurs after a pulmonary embolism and in left ventricular failure, often with a gallop rhythm.

Chest

Diminished expansion	Diminished chest expansion occurs in chronic bronchitis and emphysema.
Right ventricular heave	A right ventricular heave may be palpable in cor pulmonale and in cyanotic congenital heart disease and the latter may be associated with a thrill.

Abdomen

Hepatosplenomegaly *Hepatomegaly*	Hepatosplenomegaly may be evident in polycythaemia rubra vera, while hepatomegaly is common in congestive cardiac failure.

PERCUSSION

Hyperresonance *Stony dullness*	Percussion of the chest may reveal hyperresonance with emphysema, dullness in pneumonic consolidation or stony dullness with a pleural effusion in pulmonary embolism or bronchial carcinoma.

AUSCULTATION

Lungs

Rhonchi	Auscultation of the chest may reveal rhonchi or wheeze in chronic bronchitis and early inspiratory crepitations due to small airway obstruction. Late inspiratory crepitations may be due to pulmonary congestion in left ventricular failure and cyanotic congenital heart disease or fibrosis, as in fibrosing alveolitis. Bronchial breathing and crepitations may be heard over pneumonic consolidation.
Crepitations	
Pleural rub	A pleural rub may be heard with pulmonary embolism or pneumonia.

Heart

Pulmonary systolic murmur	Congenital heart disease is divided into cyanotic and acyanotic varieties. In cyanotic congenital heart disease, a right-to-left shunt exists. This group includes Fallot's tetralogy, Eisenmegner's complex and transposition of the great vessels. Murmurs appropriate for these conditions should be listened for.

False Cyanosis

	Blue discolouration which simulates cyanosis occurs in methaemoglobinaemia and sulphaemoglobinaemia which are usually drug related.

13. JAUNDICE

The commonest causes of jaundice in the United Kingdom, which should be borne in mind when examining an icteric patient, are hepatitis, cirrhosis, gallstones, pancreatic carcinoma, congestion, drugs and Gilbert's disease.

INSPECTION
General

Jaundice

The presence of jaundice should be confirmed by inspecting, in good natural lighting, the sclera and skin. The frenulum of the tongue may exhibit a yellow discolouration early in hyperbilirubinaemia.

Carotenaemia

Yellow skin with white sclera may be seen in carotenaemia such as occurs in hypothyroidism, vegetarians or food faddists. Hyperbilirubinaemia can be detected as jaundice only once it has reached approximately 50 μmol/l. The severity of jaundice should be gauged. A greenish tinge due to biliverdin deposition suggests chronic jaundice as occurs in primary biliary cirrhosis or chronic extrahepatic biliary obstruction.

Pigmentation

Grey complexion
Patchy, hyper- and hypopigmentation
Vitiligo

Other abnormalities of pigmentation as well as jaundice may be present in patients with liver disease, such as the slatey-grey complexion in haemochromatosis, areas of patchy, hyper- and hypopigmentation in porphyria cutanea tarda and vitiligo in chronic active hepatitis and pernicious anaemia.

Acanthosis nigricans

Acanthosis nigricans, a brownish, thickened, velvety area of skin, especially on the back of the neck, in the axillae, perianally or in the inguinal region, in adults is associated with malignancy, particularly pancreatic.

Scratch marks	Cholestatic jaundice frequently produces pruritus, possibly due to skin deposition of bile acids. Scratch marks therefore should be sought.
Injection marks	Evidence of intravenous drug abuse should be looked for and if found, should alert one to the possibility of hepatitis B.
Weight loss	Evidence of recent weight loss may be seen in patients with liver disease and/or malignancy.

Head and Neck

Cushingoid facies	A Cushingoid appearance may occur in alcoholics or be due to steroid therapy used to treat such conditions as chronic active hepatitis.
Xanthelasma	The lids and periorbital tissue should be inspected for xanthelasmata which are associated with
Kayser-Fleischer rings	chronic cholestasis, and the eyes for Kayser-Fleischer rings of Wilson's disease.
Anaemia	The combination of anaemia and jaundice occurs with haemolysis and with gastrointestinal bleeding associated with cirrhosis or with gastrointestinal malignancy with hepatic metastases.

Examination of the remainder of the face may reveal some clues as to the cause of jaundice.

	The alcoholic frequently has a flushed appearance
Acne rosacea	with or without acne rosacea, rhinophyma, paper-
Rhinophyma	money telangiectasis, parotitis and spider naevi (see
Parotitis	Ch. 5).
JVP	A raised jugular venous pressure should be looked for as it may occur secondary to a pericardial effusion due to malignancy or with hypoalbuminaemia or in congestive cardiac failure which may cause such hepatic congestion as to cause jaundice.
Breath	The breath should be smelt for the sickly sweet odour of hepatic foetor.

Limbs

Leukonychia	The hands should be examined for leukonychia,
Finger clubbing	finger clubbing, palmar erythema, Dupuytren's
Palmar erythema	contracture and asterixis, all of which occur in liver
Dupuytren's contracture	disease.
Asterixis	
Smooth nails	Shiny smooth nails may be produced by repeated scratching.

Ankle oedema	Ankle oedema should be checked for and, if present, may suggest either hypoalbuminaemia or congestive cardiac failure.
Pyoderma gangrenosum	Pyoderma gangrenosum or erythema nodosum should alert one to the possibility of sclerosing cholangitis secondary to inflammatory bowel disease.
Thrombophlebitis	Thrombophlebitis is associated with pancreatic carcinoma.

Trunk

Gynaecomastia *Spider naevi* *Venous distention* *Ascites*	The chest and abdomen should be inspected for gynaecomastia, spider naevi, venous distention, including the rare caput medusae, and the flank distention and umbilical herniation produced by ascites.
Reduced body hair	Absent or diminished axillary and pubic hair should be looked for as a stigma of chronic liver disease.
Masses	Large abdominal masses may be visible as may cutaneous metastases.
Surgical scars	Scars of previous surgery should be identified and interpreted. A recent cholecystectomy suggests retained common bile duct stones as a cause of jaundice. Any recent surgery raises the possibility of halothane hepatitis. This usually follows exposure to multiple anaesthetics. Blood transfusions used perioperatively may have caused infective hepatitis.
Ileostomy	The presence of an ileostomy in a jaundiced patient should suggest sclerosing cholangitis complicating ulcerative colitis or hepatic metastases after resection of a colonic carcinoma.

PALPATION

Lymphadenopathy	Lymphadenopathy in the jaundiced patient occurs in infectious mononucleosis, lymphoma and other malignancies and should be identified by palpation of cervical, supraclavicular, axillary and groin lymph nodes.
Gynaecomastia	Gynaecomastia should be confirmed by identifying palpable breast tissue rather than fat.
Breast lumps	In females, the breasts, the commonest site of malignancy, should always be examined.

Abdomen

Liver size/shape/ tenderness	The abdomen should be palpated carefully paying particular attention to liver size, shape and

tenderness. Remember that cirrhotic livers may be small and non-palpable. A tender liver edge suggests hepatitis or congestion; a hard, non-tender edge with splenomegaly, cirrhosis and an irregular outline suggests metastases. Tenderness below the costal margin at the ninth rib anteriorly is associated with cholecystitis (Murphy's sign) but is not specific for gallbladder inflammation.

Gallbladder   The gallbladder should be palpated for as a cystic swelling in the right hypochondrium and if identified implies obstruction of the bile duct beyond entry of the cystic duct. Although the presence of a palpable gallbladder in a jaundiced patient is said to exclude gallstones as the cause (Courvoisier's law), it should also be remembered that an enlarged gallbladder is frequently missed on examination..

Choledochal cyst   A mass in the epigastrium in a young female with jaundice should alert the examiner to the possibility of a choledochal cyst, which affects females four times more often than males.

Pancreas   Occasionally a pancreatic carcinoma or pseudo-cyst will be palpable in the epigastrium.

Spleen   The spleen, if palpable, suggests cirrhosis, haemolytic anaemia, hereditary spherocytosis, lymphoma or infectious mononucleosis.

Genitalia   The genitalia should be examined for testicular atrophy, associated with chronic alcoholism or enlargement due to neoplasm which might also involve the liver (teratoma, lymphoma).

Rectal examination   A rectal examination is essential in the complete examination of the jaundiced patient.

PERCUSSION

Masses
Ascites   Percussion should be used to confirm enlargement of organs and the presence of masses or ascites. The latter, in a jaundiced patient, is compatible with malignancy, cirrhosis or severe right ventricular failure.

Lung fields   Percussion over the lungs should be carried out to detect areas of consolidation or effusion related to lung tumours.

AUSCULTATION

Hepatic bruit   A bruit over the liver occurs in hepatitis and primary

Lung fields

or secondary liver tumours all of which may cause jaundice.
Auscultation over the lung fields should be performed especially if abnormalities are detected on percussion or malignancy is a strong possibility.

Faeces
Urine

Examination of the jaundiced patient is incomplete without examining the colour of the stools and testing the urine for urobilinogen and conjugated bilirubin. It should be remembered that urobilinogen is colourless in fresh urine.

14. URAEMIA

Uraemia frequently develops incipiently and should always be considered whilst examining patients complaining of general malaise. Thorough examination may provide important clues as to the underlying disease process. The commonest causes of chronic renal failure in the UK are chronic glomerulonephritis, chronic pyelonephritis, diabetes mellitus and hypertension.

INSPECTION

General

Conscious level

The conscious level of the patient should be assessed and drowsiness, a common feature of advanced renal failure, noted.

Respiration

The type and rate of respiration should be noted. Deep sighing breaths suggest acidosis whereas rapid shallow breathing suggests fluid overload and cardiac failure. Hiccoughs should be noted and are a sign of advanced renal failure.

Hiccoughs

Fasciculation

Irritability, fasciculation, tremor and fits are associated with advanced uraemia.

Scratch marks

Pruritus may be a major problem in patients with chronic renal failure and scratch marks may be detected on the neck and trunk as well as the limbs.

Bruising

Easy bruising also occurs due to platelet dysfunction.

Rash

The presence of a skin rash may suggest drug hypersensitivity as a cause of renal failure.

Face/Neck

Periorbital oedema

Fluid tends to collect under the influence of gravity in tissue planes of low resistance, e.g. around the eyes during the night and ankles during the day.

Uraemic frost	Crystallisation of urea in the sweat—seen on the forehead as a 'frost'—may occur in the terminal stages of renal failure.
Complexion *Anaemia* *Jaundice*	The muddy complexion of uraemic patients should be noted if present and anaemia and jaundice looked for in the conjunctiva and sclera. Conditions that cause jaundice and uraemia include Weil's disease, Gram-negative septicaemia, drug toxicity and hypersensitivity, hepatorenal syndrome (associated with chronic liver disease) haemolytic-uraemic syndrome and incompatible blood transfusion.
Jugular venous *pressure*	The jugular venous pressure should be assessed during inspection of the neck.
Tophi	The ears should be inspected for gouty tophi and calcium deposits.
Fundi	The ocular fundi should be examined particularly for evidence of hypertension or diabetes mellitus.

Hands

Evidence of arthritis should be looked for and if present should raise the possibility of analgesic abuse.

Skin turgor	Skin turgor should be assessed by pinching the skin; this is diminished when there is a pre-renal component to the renal failure.
Nails *Brown arc*	The nails should be inspected for the distal brown arc of chronic renal failure (Lindsay's nails).
Periungual infarcts	A vasculitis such as those associated with systemic lupus erythematosus, rheumatoid arthritis or polyarteritis nodosa may be manifest by periungual infarcts.
Nail-patella syndrome	Split, deformed nails, with rudimentary patellae and iliac horns make up the nail-patellae syndrome, which is inherited as an autosomal dominant trait and associated with chronic glomerulonephritis which may lead to renal failure.
Calcium deposits	Calcium deposits under the skin may be detected in patients with long-standing renal failure on dialysis.
Fistulae	A Cimino arterio-venous fistula may have been created as a means of vascular access in patients on haemodialysis. A thrill should be present over a patent fistula.

Abdomen

In patients being treated by continuous ambulatory peritoneal dialysis, a Tenchkoff catheter will be visible penetrating the abdominal wall connected to tubing and a bag. Except during 'exchange', the peritoneum will contain approximately 2 litres of dialysis fluid, and appear swollen.

Scars
Scars of previous surgical operations should be noted as recent operations may be causally related to acute renal failure; previous renal transplants are another cause.

PALPATION
The abdomen should be carefully palpated for the following:

Kidneys

The presence of two enlarged kidneys should suggest polycystic kidneys, amyloidosis or bilateral hydronephrosis. Enlargement of only one kidney should suggest absence of the other with vicarial hypertrophy, hypernephroma or unilateral hydronephrosis. More commonly in renal failure, small kidneys are found due to chronic glomerulonephritis, pyelonephritis, or hypertension. The fact that the kidneys are impalpable does not imply they are small. Renal angle tenderness should be looked for and suggests inflammation. A transplanted kidney is usually easily palpable in one or other iliac fossa.

Bladder
A palpable bladder in a patient with renal failure implies obstruction which is most commonly prostatic in origin (in men).

Liver
Patients with chronic liver disease may develop the hepatorenal syndrome. Hepatomegaly may also be found in Weil's disease, and diabetes mellitus (fatty liver) and polycystic disease.

Spleen
Although splenomegaly may rarely be found in patients with renal failure, it is important to be able to differentiate the spleen from the left kidney (especially in clinical examinations).

Tenderness
In any patient undergoing peritoneal dialysis, abdominal tenderness is an important sign and may indicate peritonitis. Confirmation is made by identifying a cloudy dialysis effluent and by bacteriological culture.

General
Rectal examination
A rectal examination should be performed looking

for benign prostatic hypertrophy or carcinoma of prostate or rectum.

Fistula thrill
The patency of a Cimino arteriovenous fistula should be confirmed by detecting an overlying thrill.

Neuropathy
In long-standing renal failure (without dialysis), a peripheral neuropathy may occur and should be sought.

PERCUSSION

Percussion has only limited application in these patients, but should be used to confirm a pleural effusion and peritoneal fluid if these are suspected.

AUSCULTATION

Heart murmurs
Heart murmurs should be listened for, in particular 'flow' murmurs in anaemic patients.

Pericardial rub
A pericardial friction sound may be due to uraemic pericarditis or indicate an underlying connective tissue disorder (e.g. systemic lupus erythematosus).

Bruit
Patent arteriovenous fistulae should have an overlying bruit. A bruit may be heard over renal artery stenosis.

Chest bases
The presence of basal crepitations in the chest is a common manifestation of fluid overload in uraemic patients.

Blood pressure
Recording the blood pressure is an essential part in the examination and hypertension, if noted, may be primary (casual) or secondary in patients with renal failure. Postural hypotension may also occur, especially following dialysis.

Urine

The examination of a patient with renal disease is incomplete without examining the urine. A fresh (warm) sample should be tested using 'labstix' (or equivalent) for protein, blood, sugar and pH. Further biochemical analyses may be indicated in selected cases.

Protein
Blood/glucose pH

Specific gravity
The specific gravity should also be measured. The sample should then be inspected with the naked eye and the colour and clarity noted. Cloudy urine is usually infected but may be due to phosphate or oxalate crystals in alkaline urine or urate crystals in acidic urine. Crystal clear urine is unlikely to be infected. Dark urine is usually either concentrated or contains blood or haemoglobin. 'Pseudohaematuria' may be due to drugs (e.g. rifampicin), dyes,

Colour

Cells
Casts
Microorganisms

myoglobin, porphyrins and bilirubin. The urine should then be centrifuged, and the deposit inspected before the majority of the supernatant is discarded. The 'pellet' is then resuspended in the remaining urine and a drop of this 'concentrate' examined under a cover-glass microscopically, looking particularly for white and red blood cells and casts. A few hyaline casts should not be regarded as abnormal. Microorganism may be identified in unstained preparations but the presence of pus cells is a more reliable indicator of infection. If infection is suspected, bacteriological culture is essential to identify the microorganism and its antibiotic sensitivity.

15. DIABETES MELLITUS

Diabetic patients are prone to numerous complications and a complete medical examination is necessary for a full assessment to be made. However, the following approach should detect most problems. Examination should be directed towards complications of the disease and its treatment.

INSPECTION

General

Hydration

The hydration state should be noted and whether the patient is obese or has obviously lost weight.

Conscious level

The conscious level should be recorded and if the patient is confused or agitated consider hypoglycaemia, especially if associated with

Sweating
Respiration

sweating and pallor.
If the patient is breathing rapidly, or has 'air hunger' (deep, sighing inspiration and expiration), underlying acidosis should be suspected.

Eyes

Iritis rubeosa

Iritis rubeosa, new vessel formation on the iris, may lead to glaucoma.

Cataracts

Cataracts occur at a younger age in diabetic patients. The snow-flake-like deposits throughout the lens cortex that used to occur in adolescent

Fundi

diabetics are now rare. Examination of the fundus is essential and should always be carried out through dilated pupils. It is usually done at the end of the examination and the relevant abnormalities are listed in Table 3.2.

Skin

Folliculitis

Inspecting the skin may reveal folliculitis and other

Intertrigo	infections such as intertrigo.
Moniliasis	Moniliasis particularly in the groin may be noted as may fungal infections of the feet.
Lipodystrophy	Lipodystrophy—painless fat atrophy at sites of insulin injection—may be noted, particularly if older types of insulin preparations have been used.
Insulin sensitivity	Insulin sensitivity may manifest itself as tender lumps at injection sites.
Necrobiosis lipoidica	On the legs, necrobiosis lipoidica diabeticorum may be seen and is characterised by atrophy of subcutaneous collagen over the shins. The lesions are violet rings with a yellow periphery and scarring and atrophy at the centre.
Brown spots	Brown spots may also appear on the shins.
Feet	The feet should be examined for evidence of impaired circulation which tends to affect the toes first.
Ulceration	Ulceration in particular must be looked for and may be due to ischaemia and/or neuropathy.

PALPATION

Tachycardia	The radial pulse should be palpated. A tachycardia may reveal an underlying infection or hypoglycaemia.
Valsalva	Lack of beat-to-beat pulse variation during a Valsalva manoeuvre may indicate autonomic neuropathy.
Peripheral pulses	All peripheral pulses should be carefully examined and may be absent in patients with severe atherosclerosis.
Skin temperature	Skin temperature of the feet should also be noted.
Hepatomegaly	Hepatomegaly may be present in diabetic patients due to fatty infiltration.
Sensation	Light touch and pinprick sensation should be assessed and are absent in peripheral neuropathy which is usually bilateral.
Vibration *Proprioception*	Vibration sense and proprioception at the ankle may also be lost in peripheral neuropathy. Loss of sensation can be associated with ulceration over pressure points, even when pulses are present.
Ankle jerk	The ankle jerk is often absent when neuropathy is present.
Mononeuritis	A mononeuritis affecting most commonly the lateral popliteal, ulnar and oculomotor nerves may occur.

Amyotrophy	Weakness with wasting of the quadriceps, which may be assymetrical and painful, occurs in diabetic amyotrophy.

PERCUSSION

Percussion has no particular place in the examination of diabetic patients except to confirm abnormalities such as pneumonia, pleural effusions and hepatomegaly where appropriate during the examination.

AUSCULTATION

Vascular bruit	Auscultation over the carotid, femoral and popliteal arteries for bruit should be performed, especially in patients with evidence of vascular disease.
Heart *Chest*	Both the heart and lung fields should be auscultated for evidence of cardiac failure. Pneumonia occurs more often in diabetic patients and should be sought.
Blood pressure	The blood pressure should be recorded and any postural fall in pressure which occurs in autonomic neuropathy noted. Hypertension, if present, should be detected and treated accordingly.
Urinalysis	Examination of the urine for ketones and glucose is an essential part of the examination of diabetic patients. Urine and blood glucose charts should also be studied, if available.

16. THYROTOXICOSIS

Thyrotoxicosis in many cases is obvious at first glance but in others, especially the elderly, it may be manifest only by such changes as atrial fibrillation. Although the clinical diagnosis may appear obvious, it is essential to confirm it biochemically before starting anti-thyroid drug therapy. Examination of a hyperthyroid patient should be directed to confirming the diagnosis with positive typical findings and elucidating the cause.

INSPECTION

General

Hyperkinesia	Thyrotoxic patients may be hyperkinetic and constant fidgeting may be noted.
Stare	There is often a characteristic staring appearance with sharp features.
Weight loss *Sweating*	Loss of weight may be apparant as may excessive sweating
Vitiligo	Vitiligo is seen in thyrotoxicosis as well as other organ-specific auto-immune diseases.
Mental state	The patient may talk rapidly whilst their mental state may be normal, hypomanic or psychotic.

Eyes

Proptosis	Proptosis should be looked for (Ch. 3) and may be bilateral or unilateral.
Exophthalmus	Exophthalmus is recognised by a visible rim of sclera above and below the iris.
Chemosis *Corneal scarring*	Chemosis (conjunctival oedema) and corneal scarring may be noted if there is difficulty in completely closing the eyes.
Lid retraction	Lid retraction is noted when a rim of sclera is visible above the iris.
Lid lag	Lid lag should also be looked for (Ch. 3).

Globe lag	Globe lag may also be detected when the upper eyelid moves up in advance of the eye on looking up.
Ophthalmoplegia	An ophthalmoplegia, with defective movement of one or more extrinsic eye muscle, should be looked for by testing eye movements. Failure of convergence is known as Moebius' sign.

Hands

Sweaty palms	The palms are often hot and sweaty in thyrotoxicosis but cold and sweaty in simple anxiety.
Tremor	A fine tremor of the outstretched hands may be noted and a sheet of paper placed over the outstretched hand emphasises this. The tremor should be differentiated from that due to Parkinsonism, alcoholism, and familial, essential tremors (Ch. 1).
Onycholysis	The nails may exhibit onycholysis (elevation of the nail from the nail bed) and finger clubbing (thyroid achropachy) should be sought.
Clubbing	

Legs

Pretibial myxoedema	Pretibial myxoedema is sometimes seen as raised, mauve-coloured patches over the shins and is invariably associated with eye signs and often with finger clubbing. It can occur in the euthyroid state and its exact cause is uncertain.

PALPATION

Pulse

Dysrhythmias	Cardiac dysrhythmias may occur and in older people this may be the main presenting feature. Such dysrhythmias include sinus tachycardia, supraventricular tachycardia, atrial flutter, atrial fibrillation and ventricular ectopic beats.

Neck

Goitre	A goitre may be present and its shape and size may help in the diagnosis. If large and smooth Grave's disease is likely, whilst a hot nodule may appear as a solitary area of swelling or be part of a multinodular gland. Thyroid carcinoma does not usually cause thyrotoxicosis.
Nodule	
Tenderness	Tenderness over the thyroid indicates inflammation

and viral thyroiditis may be associated with transient thyrotoxicosis.

Trachea The position of the trachea should be checked to be sure it is central and retrosternal extension of the thyroid should be detected by palpation in the suprasternal notch.

Chest/Abdomen

Gynaecomastia
Hepatosplenomegaly Rarely thyrotoxicosis is associated with gynaecomastia and hepatosplenomegaly.

Muscles

A proximal myopathy, tested by assessing the ease with which the patient rises from a chair, may be associated with thyrotoxicosis as may periodic paralysis and myasthenia gravis.

PERCUSSION

Retrosternal thyroid The upper aspect of the sternum should be percussed to detect dullness due to extension of thyroid tissue retrosternally.

AUSCULTATION

Bruit A bruit over the goitre is an important sign and adds considerable weight to the clinical diagnosis of thyrotoxicosis.

Cardiac Auscultation of the heart will confirm a tachycardia and may reveal a gallop rhythm of incipient heart failure, a loud first heart sound and/or a systolic apical flow murmur associated with a hyper-dynamic circulation.

Wheezing/stridor Wheezing and inspiratory stridor may be produced by tracheal compression and should be listened for.

Blood tests

The full examination of patients with suspected thyrotoxicosis must include analysis of the blood for thyroxine and/or tri-iodothyronine levels.

17. HYPERTENSION

The examination of patients with hypertension should include an attempt to identify any underlying causes, although it should be remembered that the cause of the commonest form — essential hypertension — is unknown.
Sequelae of the disease and its treatment should also be sought.

INSPECTION

Some causes of hypertension are suggested by typical appearances.

Causes of Hypertension

Cushing's syndrome

Patients with Cushing's syndrome have a moon face, facial plethora, hirsuitism, truncal obesity with wasted limbs, striae, bruising and gonadal atrophy. Children with this syndrome also may have short stature. Long term treatment with corticosteroids has a similar effect.

Acromegaly

Acromegalic subjects frequently have coarse features with prognathia, a large tongue with large, spade-like hands and feet. Other features which may be apparent include sweating, bitemporal haemanopia and organomegaly.

Coarctation of aorta

Coarctation of the aorta may be associated with a recognisable syndrome such as Turner's or Marfan's syndrome. Look for active carotid and subclavian arterial pulsation and dilated pulsating vessels in the periscapular area.

Phaeochromocytoma

Phaeochromocytoma may occur in isolation or be associated with neurofibromatosis, parathyroid adenoma or medullary carcinoma of the thyroid (multiple endocrine adenomatosis type II and von Hippel-Lindau syndrome). Signs that may indicate such associated conditions include multiple neurofibromata, café au lait spots, axillary freckles, mucosal neurofibromata, (especially on the lips), Marfanoid habitus (in multiple endocrine adenomatosis IIB), and a goitre.

Chronic renal failure Hypertension in chronic renal failure may be primary and causally related to the renal disease or secondary. Cutaneous manifestations include a 'muddy' complexion, purpura, scratch marks, uraemic frost and vascular access sites for haemodialysis.

Effects of Hypertension

Fundi The fundi should be examined for changes seen in hypertension. The classical subdivisions are as follows:

Grade I — arterial narrowing, increased light reflex of retina.

Grade II — vessel irregularity, arterio-venous nipping.

Grade III — soft, exudates, haemorrhages (usually flame shaped).

Grade IV — the above, plus papilloedema.

However, the classification into mild (Grades I and II) or accelerated (Grades III and IV) is clinically more useful.

Cardiac failure The cardiovascular system must be examined for cardiac failure, looking for tachycardia, tachypnoea, an elevated JVP and ankle oedema (Ch. 6).

Hemiparesis Complications of hypertension such as hemiparesis may be easily recognisable.

PALPATION

Peripheral Pulses

Large volume A large volume pulse may be associated with systolic hypertension and occurs in 'high output' states (Ch. 6).

Radial-femoral delay In coarctation of the aorta, small and/or delayed femoral pulses may be present and periscapular vessels may also be palpable. Absent or reduced femoral pulses may also be found in aortic dissection.

Praecordial Palpation

Apex beat Praecordial palpation may reveal a forceful apex

Left ventricular heave	beat with or without the left ventricular heave of left ventricular hypertrophy associated with long-standing hypertension. The apex beat may be displaced laterally and/or inferiorly in left ventricular dilatation.
Double apical impulse	A palpable fourth heart sound may also be detected as a double apical impulse in this situation.
Right ventricular heave	Pulmonary hypertension leads to right ventricular hypertrophy which produces a 'right ventricular heave' which is felt to the left of the sternum.
Sacral/ankle oedema	Pitting oedema should be looked for over the anterior aspect of the tibia and over the sacrum when cardiac failure is present as a complication of hypertension.
Periorbital oedema	Periorbital puffiness occurs, particularly in children, in glomerulonephritis, an uncommon cause of hypertension.

Abdomen

Kidneys	The abdomen should be examined and the kidneys palpated. Bilateral renal enlargement is found in polycystic kidney disease while unilateral enlargement (the opposite kidney) occurs in renal artery stenosis. Most other renal conditions associated with hypertension tend to produce small shrunken kidneys (which cannot be palpated).
Adrenal tumours	Adrenal tumours resulting in hypertension (phaeochromocytoma or adrenal adenoma) are rarely palpable.

AUSCULTATION

Blood Pressure

The blood pressure must be measured (rather than relying on TPR charts at the foot of the bed), and which arm used and patient's position (erect, supine or sitting) recorded. In obese subjects, a large sphygmomanometer cuff must be used to avoid spuriously high readings. Although recording phase 5 (disappearance of Korotkoff sounds) is becoming more popular than phase 4 (muffling of sounds) as a measure of diastolic blood pressure, the latter probably more accurately reflects true intra-arterial pressure. Recording which phase (4 or 5) has been measured is to be encouraged. Checking the systolic pressure by palpation over the radial artery should prevent the mistake of starting to record the systolic pressure in the ausculating gap, an area of auscultatory silence below the systolic pressure, which exists in an occasional patient. Postural hypotension in a hypertensive patient should raise the possibility of an underlying phaeochromocytoma although more often it is related to drug therapy.

Cardiac Murmurs

Cardiac auscultation may reveal murmurs related to hypertension. Aortic regurgitation is associated with a large pulse pressure and systolic hypertension and is characterised by a blowing early diastolic murmur. Aortic or pulmonary flow murmurs may be heard in hyperdynamic states. A harsh continuous murmur radiating to the back between the scapulae with or without an aortic ejection click (bicuspid valve) may be audible in coarctation of the aorta.

Basal crepitations

Basal pulmonary crepitations in left ventricular failure are usually late inspiratory and medium pitched, and fail to clear after the patient is asked to cough. Radiological changes precede these clinical signs.

Renal bruit

Abdominal bruits are fairly common in the young and are usually innocent. The murmur of renal artery stenosis may be heard in the loins, both lateral regions and the midline. Bruits may also originate from aortic aneurysms which are associated with hypertension. Abdominal bruits, however, most commonly arise from an atheromatous aorta in patients who do not have either renal artery stenosis or an aortic aneurysm.

Effects of Therapy

Effects of therapy should be looked for and include gout, dehydration or muscle weakness (hypokalaemia) from diuretics; bradycardia, cardiac failure or cold peripheries from beta-blockers; reflex tachycardia or flushing from vasodilators; postural hypotension from methyl-dopa, prazosin and others; hypertrichosis from minoxidil; lupus erythematosus from hydralazine.

18. ATAXIA

Ataxia occurs when postural control is impaired leading to clumsy or uncoordinated movements. The two main causes are diseases of the cerebellum and of sensory nerves.

INSPECTION

Gait ataxia

Inspection of the patient's gait is essential and should be carried out first. Incoordination whilst walking is referred to as gait ataxia. Be careful to be standing nearby in case the patient should fall. As sensory ataxia can be mitigated to some extent by visual information, it is typically worse when the patient closes his eyes, whilst cerebellar ataxia is unchanged. Be careful not to misinterpret the rather hesitant gait of elderly patients who suffer from drop attacks or vertigo as ataxia. More subtle incoordination in walking should be elicited by asking the patient to walk heel-to-toe, initially with eyes open and then closed.

Romberg's sign

Rombergism should then be assessed with the patient standing with feet together. Slight or even moderate swaying is not necessarily abnormal and a positive Romberg's sign should only be recorded if the patient sways so much with their eyes closed that they would fall without support or corrective measures. Rombergism is a sign of posterior column damage. Patients with cerebellar lesions tend to lean or fall towards the side of the lesion. Such a tendency can be displayed by asking the patient to walk in circles, which become increasingly small when turning towards the side of the lesion and increasingly large in the opposite direction.

Colour

Vitiligo, pallor and lemon-yellow pigmentation may

occur in pernicious anaemia, which along with other causes of peripheral neuropathy, may cause sensory ataxia.

Eyes

Pupils	The eyes should be closely inspected for Argyll Robertson pupils and bilateral ptosis seen in tabes dorsalis.
Nystagmus	Nystagmus is coarse and jerking (maximal to the side of the lesion) or rotatory in cerebellar disease while 'ataxic' nystagmus occurs in multiple sclerosis (Ch. 3). Conjunctival and skin telangiectasia occur in the rare inherited disorder, ataxia telangiectasia.

Head

Position	Tilting of the head may be present due to cerebellar hemisphere damage or to help compensation for astigmatism.
Titubation	Tremor or titubation of the head is seen in some patients with cerebellar disease.
Alcoholism	Alcoholic facies or cutaneous stigmata of alcoholic liver disease (Ch. 13) should suggest alcohol as a cause of cerebellar disease, whilst finger clubbing may be related to a primary lung tumour with cerebellar metastases.
Myxoedema	Myxoedema may cause cerebellar degeneration and should be remembered when examining ataxic patients.
Friedreich's ataxia	Pes cavus, pes equinovarus and kyphoscoliosis should suggest Friedreich's ataxia, an autosomal recessively-inherited spinocerebellar disorder which may present in childhood or adolescence. Other
Cerebellar degeneration	degenerative conditions involving the cerebellum (e.g. olivo-pontocerebellar atrophy) occur in later life.

ACTIVE MOVEMENT

Gait ataxia	See above.
Truncal ataxia	A tendency to fall backwards whilst sitting or standing is typical of midline cerebellar lesions and referred to as truncal ataxia.
Limb ataxia	Coordination in the upper limbs should be checked systematically. First, observe the patient's fully
Hyperpronation	outstretched hands looking for hyperpronation and
Tremor	tremor of cerebellar disease and then apply and suddenly remove pressure to the outstretched arms.

Over-correction	This leads to marked over-correction of the initial position in patients with cerebellar disease. The patient should then be asked to touch the tip of his nose with the index finger of both hands in turn with the eyes open initially and then closed.
Intention tremor	An intention tremor, a tremor of increasing amplitude as the hand reaches the target, is typical of cerebellar disease. A more subtle test of coordination involves asking the patient to touch first the tip of his nose and then the examiner's finger which is moved in various directions. Overshooting the target or past pointing (dysmetria)
Past pointing	is typical of cerebellar lesions. Coordination in the legs can be assessed by asking the patient to run the right foot slowly and accurately up the front of their left shin to the knee and vice versa.

Rapid Simple Movements

Dysdiadochokinesia	Dysdiadochokinesia, the inability to perform rapid simple alternating movements, should be assessed. The most usual method of checking for this is to ask the patient to tap one hand as fast as possible on the back of the other and vice versa. The same test can be used for the feet, usually asking the patient to tap their foot rapidly against the examiner's hand. Rapid alternating pronation and supination at the wrist is a further test for dysdiadochokinesia. These tests tend to be performed better on the dominant side and this should always be checked. Unilateral incoordination or ataxia can easily be identified using these tests. Be careful not to over-interpret mild bilateral incoordination. The patient's writing should also be observed as it tends to become larger (cf. Parkinsonism) and more untidy in patients with cerebellar disease.

Passive Movement

Tone	Tone should be assessed at the wrists, elbows, knees and ankles. Reduced tone, particularly if unilateral, is suggestive of ipsilateral cerebellar disease. Acute pyramidal lesions can also cause hypotonia and should be excluded.

Reflexes

Pendular

The tendon reflexes should be elicited. In peripheral neuropathy they will be absent, whilst in cerebellar disease they tend to be slower and 'pendular'.

Delayed relaxation

Delayed relaxation of the reflexes occurs in hypothyroidism, which may be the cause of cerebellar ataxia.

Plantar reflexes

The plantar reflexes should be checked and may be dorsiflexor and associated with absent ankle jerks in subacute combined degeneration, diabetes mellitus, Friedreich's ataxia, taboparesis and motor neurone disease. All but the last may cause ataxia.

Sensation

Fine touch and proprioception

Fine touch and proprioception should be checked to exclude a sensory neuropathy, causes of which include diabetes mellitus, pernicious anaemia, alcoholism and carcinomatous neuropathy.

Speech

Staccato

The quality of the patient's speech should be assessed. In cerebellar disease, it tends to be 'staccato'. Rapid repetition of words such as 'cat' or 'tick-tock' may make this obvious.

Scanning

Multiple sclerosis may cause 'scanning' speech due to combined cerebellar and pyramidal lesions. The patient should be asked if they are epileptic and/or taking phenytoin, since this may cause ataxia with high blood levels.

FURTHER EXAMINATION

Fundoscopy

Evidence of raised intracranial pressure due to a posterior fossa lesion should be sought at fundoscopy. Optic atrophy and retinal pigmentation may be due to Refsum's disease, an autosomal recessive disorder which may cause ataxia in association with deafness, muscular atrophy and peripheral neuropathy.

If the results of the examination suggest that the ataxia may be related to a carcinoma, the primary should be sought, the commonest being a bronchial carcinoma.

19. ARTHRITIS

Arthritis is a common disorder and arthritic patients are frequently used in clinical examinations. There are numerous causes of arthritis and more than one disease process may be present in an individual patient (e.g. septic monoarthritis in a patient with rheumatoid disease).

INSPECTION

Sex

The sex of the patient is important and influences the differential diagnosis of rheumatic diseases: Reiter's disease, gout and ankylosing spondylitis are much commoner in men whilst systemic lupus erythematosus, systemic sclerosis and rheumatoid arthritis are commoner in women.

Face

Cushingoid
Alopecia
Butterfly rash
Heliotrope rash

Malnourished
Gouty tophi

Cushingoid facies may be related to steroid treatment, whilst alopecia and a 'butterfly rash' occur in systemic lupus erythematosus.
A heliotrope rash of the cheeks and forehead (and knuckles) occurs in dermatomyositis.
Malnourishment may mean underlying tuberculosis.
Gouty tophi should be looked for around the cartilage of the ear.

Eyes

Anaemia
Uveitis

Dry eyes

Cataracts

The eyes should be inspected for the conjunctival pallor of anaemia and uveitis in juvenile rheumatoid arthritis, ankylosing spondylitis, Behçet's and Reiter's syndromes.
Dry eyes occur with Sjögren's syndrome and occasionally scleromalacia in rheumatoid arthritis.
Cataracts may be due to steroid or chloroquine therapy.

Mouth

Systemic sclerosis Tightening of the skin around the mouth, frequently associated with telangiectasia, occurs in systemic sclerosis.

Xerostomia Xerostomia (dry mouth) is seen in Sjögren's syndrome, while buccal ulceration is seen in Behçet's syndrome and inflammatory bowel disease.

Skin

Rashes Rashes should be looked for specifically and in good light as they are sometimes difficult to see, especially if fading. They frequently represent drug hypersensitivity but also occur in juvenile rheumatoid arthritis, rheumatic fever, secondary syphilis, brucellosis, and Henoch-Schönlein purpura. In gonococcal septicaemia, skin lesions on the periphery may be papular, pustular, haemorrhagic or necrotic.

Psoriasis The skin eruption and nail pitting of psoriasis must not be missed (Ch. 1).

Erythema marginatum Erythema marginatum may occur in rheumatic fever.

Erythema nodosum Erythema nodosum appearing as tender red nodules over the shins may accompany polyarteritis nodosa, rheumatoid arthritis, rheumatic fever, sarcoidosis, mycoplasmal infection and drug hypersensitivity, all of which may cause an arthritis.

Livedo reticularis Livedo reticularis, a reticulate pattern of skin marking similar to erythema ab igni ('Granny's tartan') is associated with polyarteritis nodosa and systemic lupus erythematosus.

Purpura Purpura may be seen in Henoch-Schönlein purpura and in thrombocytopenia, secondary to treatment (gold, penicillamine) in rheumatoid arthritis.

Ecchymoses Ecchymoses may be seen with steroid therapy and in scurvy and bleeding can affect large joints (hips and knees). Haemarthroses may occur in haemophilia but there are usually few external signs of bleeding.

Scars Scars of previous orthopaedic surgery should be noted, as should multiple abnormal scars or enterostomies, suggestive of inflammatory bowel disease.

Pigmentation Skin pigmentation may be seen in Whipple's

disease, along with lymphadenopathy, pyrexia and a migratory polyarthritis. The latter is frequently the first symptom of the disorder.

Genitalia

Ulceration
Urethral discharge
Circinate balanitis

Genital ulceration occurs in Behcet's syndrome, while urethral discharge occurs in gonorrhoea and Reiter's syndrome where circinate balanitis also may be noted.

Joints

All major joints should be inspected and compared with the opposite side looking for
1) Swelling
2) Erythema
3) Deformity
4) Associated abnormalities such as bursitis, muscle wasting and rheumatoid nodules.
The hands, elbows and feet in particular must be carefully examined. The pattern of joint involvement in different diseases is outlined in Table 19.1. A single red, swollen painful joint in a patient with a chronic arthritis may signal infection of the joint.

Hands (see Ch. 1)

Clubbing

Finger clubbing may occur in Whipple's and chronic inflammatory bowel disease, both of which may have joint manifestations, and in hypertrophic pulmonary osteoarthropathy associated with pulmonary suppuration and tumours.

Nail fold infarcts

Nail fold infarcts are seen in active rheumatoid arthritis and dermatomyositis.

Raynaud's phenomenon

Raynaud's phenomenon and sclerodactyly are features of systemic sclerosis, while subcutaneous calcified nodules in addition in the hands suggest CRST syndrome (calcinosis, Raynaud's sclerodactyly, telangectasia).

Heberden's nodes
Bouchard's nodes

Gouty tophi

Exostoses such as Heberden's nodes (distal interphalangeal joints) and Bouchard's nodes (proximal interphalangeal joints) are seen in osteoarthrosis, whilst gouty tophi (with deformity of hands if chronic) in the arthropathy of gout. Rheumatoid arthritis tends to produce ulnar deviation of the fingers and subluxation at the metacarpophalangeal joints is typical, as are 'swan-neck' and 'boutonièrre' deformities of fingers, which are due to tendon damage. Oedema of the hands

Deformities

Muscle wasting	and muscle wasting are also frequently seen in rheumatoid arthritis, which tends to cause spindle-shaped swollen fingers and spares the distal interphalangeal joints, unlike osteoarthritis and psoriasis (see Table 19.1).

Elbows

Nodules	Subcutaneous rheumatoid nodules are frequently found at the elbow and should be looked for specifically. The rheumatic nodule of acute rheumatic fever is characteristically found over the back of the skull.
Bursitis	Olecranon bursitis should be looked for (in rheumatoid arthritis, ankylosing spondylitis, gout),
Deformity	as well as deformity.
Psoriasis	Psoriatic plaques are frequently found on the elbow (e.g. the extensor surfaces).

Feet

Rheumatoid arthritis	Characteristic deformity of the feet and toes is seen in rheumatoid arthritis with dorsal subluxation of the toes exposing the metatasal heads to pressure during walking, which may lead to ulceration. Hallux valgus also typically develops.
Gout	The swollen, red, tender, painful great toe typical of an acute attack of gout should not be missed nor confused with an inflamed bunion.
Keratoderma blenorrhagica	The soles of the feet must be inspected for keratoderma blenorrhagica, the lesions of which appear initially as vesicles and later as sterile pustules with hyperkeratosis. If this is found the other features of Reiter's disease (conjunctivitis, uveitis, urethritis, circinate balanitis, mouth ulcers and Achilles' tendonitis) must be looked for.
Ankle oedema	Ankle oedema may be a feature of nephrotic syndrome related to gold and penicillamine therapy.
Leg ulcers	Leg ulcers may complicate the vasculitis of active rheumatoid arthritis.

Posture

Pelvic tilt	Abnormalities of posture may be due to arthritic processes. Tilting of the pelvis may suggest underlying osteoarthosis or rheumatoid arthritis of the hip. There will often be a compensatory scoliosis.

Table 19.1 Typical joint distribution and associated features of various arthritides.

RHEUMATOID ARTHRITIS (RA)

Hands (MCP & PIP), feet, wrists, knees, shoulders, ankles, hips, cervical spine, temperomandibular joint. Symmetrical, polyarticular nodules, muscle wasting.

Assoc. leg ulcers, scleritis, Sjögren's syndrome, vasculitis, valve and myocardial lesions, pleural effusions, alveolitis, lymphadenopathy, splenomegaly, carpal tunnel syndrome, neuropathy, anaemia, amyloid.

JUVENILE RHEUMATOID ARTHRITIS

Joints as RA—less symmetrical, sometimes monoarticular.

Assoc. lymphadenopathy, splenomegaly, pericarditis, rash, iritis, anaemia, growth retardation.

OSTEOARTHROSIS

Hands (DIP & PIP), thumb, spine, knees, hips. Polyarticular symmetrical.

Assoc. Heberden's (DIP) and Bouchard's (PIP) joints (osteophytes).

REITER'S SYNDROME

Knees, ankles, feet (MTP), sacro-iliitis. Polyarticular asymmetrical.

Assoc. urethritis, balanitis, keratoderma blenorrhagica, conjunctivitis, calcaneal spurs, plantar fasciitis.

ANKYLOSING SPONDYLITIS

Sacro-iliitis, spine, ribs, also hips, knees, ankles.

Assoc. uveitis, aortic incompetence, alveolitis.

GOUT

Great toe (MTP), hands (DIP, PIP), gouty tophi. Asymmetrical, oligoarticular. (Negatively birefringent needle shaped urate crystals.)

PSEUDOGOUT

Knees, other large joints. Asymmetrical, oligarticular (positively birefringent brick-shaped pyrophosphate crystals), idiopathic or in haemachromatosis, hyperparathyroidism, acromegaly.

PSORIASIS

Hands (DIP) especially, may simulate RA; sacroliitis.

Assoc. Nail pitting, psoriatic rash (elbows and knees).

SYSTEMIC LUPUS ERYTHEMATOSUS

Joints as RA (less deformity). Symmetrical, polyarticular.

Assoc. rash, renal failure, pericarditis, cardiac lesions, pleurisy, pulmonary fibrosis, neuropathy, fits, psychosis.

SYSTEMIC SCLEROSIS

Fingers especially, symmetrical.

Assoc. skin bound down, oedematous and smooth, telangiectasia, ulceration, renal failure, Raynaud's and Sjögren's syndromes.

MCP = metacarpophalangeal; PIP = proximal interphalangeal;
DIP = distal interphalangeal; MTP = metatarsophalangeal.

Knee	A genu valgum deformity may complicate a deforming knee arthropathy.
Spine	In ankylosing spondylitis a characteristic fixed stooped posture may be noted.

PALPATION

Joints	After inspection, the joints should be palpated. Enquire of the patient whether any joint is tender before proceeding and handle with care. There is not time, particularly during an examination to palpate all joints and special attention should therefore be directed to deformed and swollen joints.
Tenderness	The degree of tenderness should be assessed as well as soft tissue swelling. Calcaneal tenderness is noted in Reiter's syndrome and ankylosing spondylitis.
Nodules	Rheumatoid nodules along the radius may be missed on inspection and should be sought specifically by palpation.
Effusions	Joint effusions may be identified clinically and should be looked for particularly in the knee. Conditions which may simulate a knee effusion are prepatellar bursitis and cellulitis.
Patella tap	Tests used to detect presence of fluid in the knee joint include the patella tap where the patella can be bounced off underlying bone once fluid in the suprapatellar pouch is diverted into the knee joint by manual compression. This test identifies moderate volumes. Smaller volumes can be identified by pressing over the hollow on one side of the patella and watching for filling of the opposite hollow. Large volumes are usually obvious, but can be confirmed by transmitting a fluid impulse from around the ligamentum patellae below the patella to the swelling above the patella.
Hip	In osteoartherosis of the hip, there may be apparent shortening of the leg and measuring the distance from the medial malleolus to the anterior superior iliac spine will help differentiate from true shortening. Thomas' test will reveal flexion deformity i.e. flexion of the unaffected hip straightens the lumbar spine and leads to elevation of the affected leg.

Movement

Active/passive	Joints should be put through their range of

movements initially actively (by the patient) and then passively, and the degree of movement recorded.

Hypermobility
Hypermobility of joints should be looked for, particularly of the fingers and wrist, and occurs in Marfan's or Ehlers-Danlos syndrome, osteogenesis imperfecta, and homocystinuria. It may also be idiopathic or associated with deformity as in rheumatoid arthritis or Charcot's joints (grossly disordered painless joints seen in the knee and ankle in tabes dorsalis and diabetes mellitus and in the arm in syringomyelia).

Crepitus
Instability should be looked for during passive joint manipulation. Crepitus may be felt during movement of damaged joints.

Flexion, extension and rotation of the spine should be included if ankylosing spondylitis is not to be missed, and sacro-iliac joint tenderness (on springing the pelvis) may be seen early in ankylosing spondylitis and Reiter's syndrome.

Abdomen

Splenomegaly
The abdomen should be palpated in patients with evidence of rheumatoid disease, looking specifically for the splenomegaly of Felty's syndrome and juvenile rheumatoid arthritis.

PERCUSSION
Percussion is of limited value in examining patients with joint disease, except in identifying areas of tenderness over the spine (percussing with the ulnar aspect of the clenched fist), and in detecting pleural effusions, which occur in systemic lupus erythematosus and rheumatoid disease.

AUSCULTATION
Creaking and clicking during movement of damaged joints is often audible without the stethoscope.

Heart murmurs
Cardiac auscultation may detect cardiac murmurs in acute rheumatic fever (Carey Coombs), ankylosing spondylitis and tertiary syphilis (aortic

Pericardial rub
regurgitation). A pericardial rub may be heard in rheumatoid disease and systemic lupus

Crepitations
erythematosus whilst pulmonary crepitations occur in ankylosing spondylitis (apical) and rheumatoid disease, systemic lupus erythematosus and sarcoidosis (basal).

INDEX